Patient Safety

Editors

DAVID W. TODD
JEFFREY D. BENNETT

ORAL AND MAXILLOFACIAL SURGERY CLINICS OF NORTH AMERICA

www.oralmaxsurgery.theclinics.com

Consulting Editor
RICHARD H. HAUG

May 2017 • Volume 29 • Number 2

ELSEVIER

1600 John F. Kennedy Boulevard • Suite 1800 • Philadelphia, Pennsylvania, 19103-2899

http://www.oralmaxsurgery.theclinics.com

ORAL AND MAXILLOFACIAL SURGERY CLINICS OF NORTH AMERICA Volume 29, Number 2
May 2017 ISSN 1042-3699, ISBN-13: 978-0-323-52854-2

Editor: John Vassallo; j.vassallo@elsevier.com
Developmental Editor: Colleen Dietzler

Oral and Maxillofacial Surgery Clinics of North America (ISSN 1042-3699) is published quarterly by Elsevier Inc., 360 Park Avenue South, New York, NY 10010-1710. Months of issue are February, May, August, and November. Business and Editorial Offices: 1600 John F. Kennedy Blvd., Suite 1800, Philadelphia, PA 19103-2899. Periodicals postage paid at New York, NY and additional mailing offices. Subscription prices are $385.00 per year for US individuals, $653.00 per year for US institutions, $100.00 per year for US students and residents, $455.00 per year for Canadian individuals, $783.00 per year for Canadian institutions, $520.00 per year for international individuals, $783.00 per year for international institutions and $235.00 per year for Canadian and foreign students/residents. To receive student/resident rate, orders must be accompanied by name or affiliated institution, date of term, and the *signature* of program/residency coordinator on institution letterhead. Orders will be billed at individual rate until proof of status is received. Foreign air speed delivery is included in all *Clinics* subscription prices. All prices are subject to change without notice. **POSTMASTER:** Send address changes to *Oral and Maxillofacial Surgery Clinics of North America,* Elsevier Periodicals **Customer Service, 11830 Westline Industrial Drive, St. Louis, MO 63146. Tel: 1-800-654-2452 (U.S. and Canada); 314-447-8871 (outside U.S. and Canada). Fax: 314-447-8029. E-mail: journals customerservice-usa@elsevier.com (for print support); journalsonlinesupport-usa@elsevier.com (for online support)**.

Reprints. For copies of 100 or more, of articles in this publication, please contact the Commercial Reprints Department, Elsevier Inc., 360 Park Avenue South, New York, NY 10010-1710. Tel.: 212-633-3874; Fax: 212-633-3820; Email: reprints@elsevier.com.

Oral and Maxillofacial Surgery Clinics of North America is covered in *MEDLINE/PubMed (Index Medicus)*, *Science Citation Index Expanded (SciSearch®)*, *Journal Citation Reports/Science Edition*, and *Current Contents®/Clinical Medicine*.

Contributors

CONSULTING EDITOR

RICHARD H. HAUG, DDS
Professor and Chief, Oral Maxillofacial Surgery, Carolinas Medical Center, Charlotte, North Carolina

EDITORS

DAVID W. TODD, DMD, MD, FACD
Private Practice, Lakewood, New York; UPMC Chautauqua WCA Hospital, Jamestown, New York

JEFFREY D. BENNETT, DMD
Indianapolis, Illinois

AUTHORS

SHELLY ABRAMOWICZ, DMD, MPH
Assistant Professor, Division of Oral and Maxillofacial Surgery, Department of Surgery, Emory University School of Medicine, Children's Healthcare of Atlanta, Atlanta, Georgia

LEON A. ASSAEL, DMD
Professor and Dean Emeritus, Division of Oral and Maxillofacial Surgery, Department of Developmental and Surgical Sciences, University of Minnesota, Minneapolis, Minnesota

JEFFREY D. BENNETT, DMD
Indianapolis, Illinois

ROBERT C. BOSACK, DDS
Private Practice, Clinical Assistant Professor, College of Dentistry, University of Illinois at Chicago, Orland Park, Illinois

KEVIN J. BUTTERFIELD, MD, DDS
Chief, Division of Dentistry/Oral and Maxillofacial Surgery, Assistant Professor, Department of Otolaryngology, Ottawa Hospital, University of Ottawa School of Medicine, Ottawa, Ontario, Canada

LISAMARIE DI PASQUALE, DDS, MD
Resident, Division of Oral and Maxillofacial Surgery, Department of Craniofacial Sciences, University of Connecticut, Farmington, Connecticut

ELIE M. FERNEINI, DMD, MD, MHS, MBA, FACS
Private Practice, Greater Waterbury Oral and Maxillofacial Surgery, Medical Director, Beau Visage Med Spa, Cheshire, Connecticut; Assistant Clinical Professor, Division of Oral and Maxillofacial Surgery, Department of Craniofacial Sciences, University of Connecticut, Farmington, Connecticut

KATHERINE A. KEELEY, DDS, MD
Private Practice, Henderson, Nevada; Vice Chief Medical Officer, Sunrise Hospital and Medical Center, Clinical Instructor, Department of Surgery, University of Nevada School of Medicine, Las Vegas, Nevada

KYLE J. KRAMER, DDS, MS
Assistant Clinical Professor, Department of Oral Surgery and Hospital Dentistry, Indiana University School of Dentistry, Indianapolis, Indiana

JAROM E. MAUER, DMD
Private Practice, Eastern Iowa Oral and
Maxillofacia Surgery, Cedar Rapids, Iowa

JUSTINE S. MOE, DDS, MD
Resident, Division of Oral and Maxillofacial
Surgery, Department of Surgery, Emory
University School of Medicine, Atlanta, Georgia

RICHARD M. RITT, EMT-P, MA
President, Consultant Dental Simulation
Specialists Inc, Kildeer, Illinois

STEVEN M. ROSER, DMD, MD
Hill Chair and Professor of Oral and Maxillofacial
Surgery, Department of Surgery, Emory
University School of Medicine, Atlanta, Georgia

DANIEL S. SARASIN, DDS
Private Practice, Cedar Rapids Oral Surgery
and Implant Center, Cedar Rapids, Iowa

JAMES Q. SWIFT, DDS, FACS
Professor and Program Director, Advanced
Specialty Education in Oral and Maxillofacial
Surgery, Division of Oral and Maxillofacial
Surgery, University of Minnesota, Minneapolis,
Minnesota

DAVID W. TODD, DMD, MD, FACD
Private Practice, Lakewood, New York;
UPMC Chautauqua WCA Hospital,
Jamestown, New York

Contents

Preface   ix

David W. Todd and Jeffrey D. Bennett

General Concepts of Patient Safety for the Oral and Maxillofacial Surgeon   121

David W. Todd

Whether managing patients in private offices or as part of a care team at hospitals, oral and maxillofacial surgeons owe it to patients to understand medical error and take action to reduce its frequency and adverse effects. This article reviews general concepts of patient safety, including high-reliability organization, crew resource management, simulation training, root cause analysis, and just culture.

Preoperative Preparation and Planning of the Oral and Maxillofacial Surgery Patient   131

Jeffrey D. Bennett

Every patient is different and has the potential to respond unfavorably to anesthetic and surgical intervention. Preparation is the key to optimizing patient outcome.

Proper Management of Medications to Limit Errors: What the Oral Surgeon Should Know to Limit Medication Errors and Adverse Drug Events   141

Daniel S. Sarasin and Jarom E. Mauer

Providing safe and effective ambulatory anesthesia is a key component in delivering optimal care to oral and maxillofacial patients. Unfortunately, medication errors and adverse drug events (ADEs) occur in offices, as they do in hospital operating rooms. Preparing and delivering medication seems simple. In reality, this is a complex process with multiple opportunities for drug errors leading to actual or potential ADEs. This article reviews medication errors and ADEs, introduces a medication safety paradigm for oral and maxillofacial surgery facilities, and provides practical safety initiatives that can be implemented to achieve the goal of optimal anesthesia patient care and safety.

Preventing Wrong-Site Surgery in Oral and Maxillofacial Surgery   151

Leon A. Assael

This article discusses the risk for wrong-site surgery in oral and maxillofacial surgery and the development and utility of checklists. The intent of checklists and the specific applicability of each of them to ambulatory oral and maxillofacial surgery are presented. Checklists and other considerations to mitigate the risk of wrong-site surgery are evaluated. The role of interprofessional teams in improving patient care outcomes with the checklist as a vehicle is evaluated. Recommendations for the use of checklists and related methods in the ambulatory oral and maxillofacial surgery setting are made.

Monitoring for the Oral and Maxillofacial Surgeon   159

Robert C. Bosack

Parenteral medications are titrated in the oral and maxillofacial surgery office to achieve moderate sedation, deep sedation, or general anesthesia while continuously maintaining spontaneous ventilation with an open airway. After initial drug administration, the provider assesses and interprets both the level of anesthesia and the presence/severity of adverse side effects, both of which guide further drug titration, cessation, reversal, or medical management. This assessment is called monitoring, which guides the conduct of anesthesia delivery and becomes the essence of this art.

Simulation Training for the Office-Based Anesthesia Team   169

Richard M. Ritt, Jeffrey D. Bennett, and David W. Todd

An OMS office is a complex environment. Within such an environment, a diverse scope of complex surgical procedures is performed with different levels of anesthesia, ranging from local anesthesia to general anesthesia, on patients with varying comorbidities. Optimal patient outcomes require a functional surgical and anesthetic team who are familiar with both standard operational principles and emergency recognition and management. Offices with high volume and time pressure add further stress and potential risk to the office environment. Creating and maintaining a functional surgical and anesthetic team that is competent with a culture of patient safety and risk reduction is a significant challenge that requires time, commitment, planning, and dedication. This article focuses on the role of simulation training in office training and preparation.

Fire Safety for the Oral and Maxillofacial Surgeon and Surgical Staff   179

LisaMarie Di Pasquale and Elie M. Ferneini

Fire in the operating room is a life-threatening emergency that demands quick, efficient intervention. Because the circumstances surrounding fires are generally well-understood, virtually every operating room fire is preventable. Before every operating room case, thorough preprocedure "time outs" should address each team members' awareness of specific fire risks and agreement regarding fire concerns and emergency actions. Fire prevention centers on 3 constituent parts of the fire triad necessary for fire formation. Regular fire drills should guide policies and procedures to prevent surgical fires. Delivering optimal patient care in emergent situations requires surgical team training, practicing emergency roles, and specific actions.

Outpatient Anesthetic Safety Considerations for Obstructive Sleep Apnea   189

Kevin J. Butterfield

Most patients with obstructive sleep apnea (OSA) are not diagnosed preoperatively. The STOP-Bang questionnaire may identify patients at risk of OSA, especially those with severe OSA. Patients with mild to moderate OSA, with optimized comorbidities, can usually safely undergo outpatient surgery. Patients with severe OSA, who are not optimized medically, should avoid outpatient surgery.

Discharge Criteria, Impact of the Patient and the Procedure: What the Oral Surgeon Should Know   197

Kyle J. Kramer

This article is a concise review of discharge criteria following sedation or anesthesia relevant to the oral and maxillofacial surgeon. Topics covered include a general overview of the need for objective discharge criteria, a review of standardized criteria, and a brief discussion on specific anesthetic, patient, and surgical factors that can impact the safety of the immediate postoperative recovery and postdischarge periods.

Equipment Safety, Maintenance and Inspection: What the Oral Surgeon Needs to Know   209

Katherine A. Keeley

> Many oral and maxillofacial surgical procedures are done in an office-based setting, with many oral and maxillofacial surgeons involved in oversight of equipment maintenance. Goals in equipment management are to prevent harm to patients and staff, stay compliant with current regulations, and increase equipment longevity. This article covers the safety, maintenance, and inspection related to electrical equipment used in the treatment of patients, autoclaves, radiograph machines, nitrous oxide and oxygen medical gases, and required back-up power and lighting. An office should always follow manufacturer's recommendations regarding maintenance and inspection and document policies and monitoring so compliance can be assured.

Patient Safety and the Malpractice System   223

James Q. Swift

> The cost of health care in the United States and malpractice insurance has escalated greatly over the past 30 years. In an ideal world, the goals of the tort system would be aligned with efforts at improving safety. In fact, there is little evidence that the tort system and the processes of risk management and informed consent have improved patient safety. This article explores the disunion between patient safety and the malpractice system.

Quality Improvement and Reporting Systems: What the Oral and Maxillofacial Surgeon Should Know   229

Justine S. Moe, Shelly Abramowicz, and Steven M. Roser

> Health care is an inherently dangerous environment, and patient safety should be an explicit goal of oral and maxillofacial surgery. Important components of a safety program include a nonpunitive safety culture, the implementation of patient safety practices, standardized incident reporting and adverse event analysis, regular self-assessment, and internal and external benchmarking. Implementation of a safety program requires the strong commitment of leadership and the engagement and empowerment of all employees. Oral and maxillofacial surgery can become the model dental specialty by implementing patient safety programs for office-based surgery. The programs could then be used by all dental practitioners performing oral surgery in the office.

Index   239

ORAL AND MAXILLOFACIAL SURGERY CLINICS OF NORTH AMERICA

FORTHCOMING ISSUES

August 2017
Evaluation of the Surgical Margin
Joshua Lubek and Kelly Magliocca, *Editors*

November 2017
Controversies in Oral and Maxillofacial Surgery
Luis G. Vega and Daniel J. Meara, *Editors*

February 2018
Pediatric TMJ Disorders
Shelly Abramowicz, *Editor*

RECENT ISSUES

February 2017
Emerging Biomaterials and Techniques in Tissue Regeneration
Alan S. Herford, *Editor*

November 2016
Coagulopathy
Jeffrey D. Bennett, Elie M. Ferneini, *Editors*

August 2016
Oral and Maxillofacial Pain
Steven J. Scrivani, *Editor*

THE CLINICS ARE NOW AVAILABLE ONLINE!
Access your subscription at:
www.theclinics.com

Preface

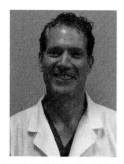

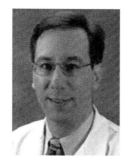

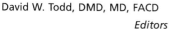

David W. Todd, DMD, MD, FACD   Jeffrey D. Bennett, DMD

Editors

The Oral and Maxillofacial Surgeon (OMS) faces many challenges in providing excellent patient treatment. Like other health care providers, OMSs want to *help* their patients. Most importantly, OMSs desire *to do no harm* to their patients in the process of administering care. Simply put, patient safety is the basis for good patient care. Patient safety must be thoughtfully and purposefully addressed to minimize adverse outcomes in delivering care to our patients. Patient safety involves multiple disciplines. Unlike large institutions, many OMSs are in private practices, and even the largest OMS groups do not have risk managers, compliance officers, medical directors, and quality officers to address the myriad of possible patient safety concerns, yet it should be expected that they maintain the same level of patient safety.

This issue is dedicated to patient safety in the field of oral and maxillofacial surgery. The various topics included in this issue address the specific areas of concern in our field. The reader will see that many areas of concern overlap with other areas of medicine quite well. The most important concept embodied in this issue is the recognition that human error occurs in the best trained and dedicated health care professionals, and taking steps to recognize, minimize, and intercept these errors is the key to reducing the likelihood of error and minimizing the impact of adverse events.

Health care is evolving. Many of us have expanded our practice beyond what we were taught as students and residents. The old adage that *it has always been done that way* is simply unacceptable. Oral and maxillofacial surgery prides itself on the scope and quality of care that its practitioners provide. It is our sincere hope that the reader will review these concepts of patient safety and take steps to implement a program to enhance the culture of safety in their offices.

David W. Todd, DMD, MD, FACD
Private Practice
120 Southwestern Drive
Lakewood, NY 14750, USA

Jeffrey D. Bennett, DMD
1481 West 10th Street
Indianapolis, IN 46202, USA

E-mail addresses:
david@dwtodd.com (D.W. Todd)
jb2omfs@gmail.com (J.D. Bennett)

Oral Maxillofacial Surg Clin N Am 29 (2017) ix
http://dx.doi.org/10.1016/j.coms.2017.03.001
1042-3699/17/© 2017 Published by Elsevier Inc.

General Concepts of Patient Safety for the Oral and Maxillofacial Surgeon

CrossMark

David W. Todd, DMD, MD, FACD

KEYWORDS

- Patient safety • High-reliability organization • Crew resource management • Simulation training
- Root cause analysis • Medical error • Adverse event • Just culture

KEY POINTS

- Patient safety is an important concept for the oral and maxillofacial surgeon in all clinical settings and is the basis for good patient care.
- Medical error is pervasive in health care and preventing medical error is a complex process involving many disciplines.
- Understanding various types of medical errors allows for identification of training, processes, and checklists to help reduce the likelihood of medical error.
- Following principles of high-reliability organizations and simulation training should allow for a reduction in medical error.

An aircraft carrier deck is among the most dangerous work environments imaginable (**Fig. 1**). Jet aircraft are launched and retrieved, often simultaneously; live ordnance is loaded onto and off of aircraft; jet fuel is loaded into aircraft; jet blast and propellers are threats; and catapults are continuously in action on a moving surface in all weather conditions, both during the day and night. The multiple aircraft have different munitions, load requirements, restrictions, and different catapult settings.

The men and women who work on the aircraft carrier deck are highly trained, work in teams with color-coded vests, know their roles extremely well, and most often have only a high school education and technical training for the tasks that they perform. Communication is scripted, precise, and limited to roles that are well-described and rehearsed. There is a hierarchy of command that oversees the functions on the deck of the aircraft carrier. The safety record of aircraft carriers is very good and the US Navy has developed

systems, teams, procedures, and checklists to make its ability to carry out its mission highly reliable. Similar systems are in place in other branches of the military, in the aviation industry, and the nuclear industry in which high-risk operations are carried out with similar excellent safety records. These organizations and their approaches to operations are called high-reliability organizations (HROs). See later discussion of the characteristics of HROs. Unfortunately, most health care organizations, from private offices to large hospitals, do not exhibit the characteristics of an HRO, quality of care and safety of care provided is variable, and many errors occur routinely.

Primum non nocere, first do no harm, has been a guiding principle in medicine since Hippocrates time. Those who decide to go into health care have a desire to help patients using their chosen specialty. This article is dedicated to an overview of patient safety. Why is it important to explore this topic as a health care provider? First, patient safety is the basis for good patient care. When

The author has no financial interests in any company or product and has no disclosures.
Private Practice, Oral and Maxillofacial Surgery, 120 Southwestern Drive, Lakewood, NY 14750, USA
E-mail address: david@dwtodd.com

Oral Maxillofacial Surg Clin N Am 29 (2017) 121–129
http://dx.doi.org/10.1016/j.coms.2016.12.001

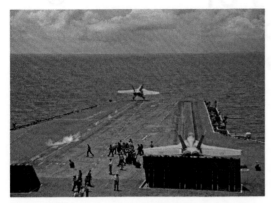

Fig. 1. Flight deck of a US aircraft carrier. (*From* Department of the Navy. Available at: http://www.navy.mil/management/photodb/photos/160719-N-YB023-018.JPG. Accessed July 20, 2016.)

patients seek medical or dental care, it is most important that patients are not harmed in the process of receiving care. Second, this topic is important because most health care professionals do not have formal training and practice in patient safety. Third, it is a complex topic that involves multiple disciplines outside of health care that are explored in this brief introduction (see discussion of details, in this issue). Finally, patient safety is an evolving topic and clinicians are currently in the second phase of development, whereby the low-hanging fruit has been harvested and real gains in measurable patient safety require more research, measurement, and practice to realize the goal of reducing patient harm in the United States and across the globe.

Health care is a complex task requiring history taking, examination, laboratory data and imaging interpretation, diagnosis, communication among different providers and care givers, patient education, medical or surgical treatment, and follow-up. A signature realization in the 1990s was that, despite all the advances in modern medicine, medical care was fraught with error and adverse events. Through thousands of chart reviews in 3 different states, the US Institute of Medicine (IOM) was able to calculate that 44,000 to 98,000 Americans die each year from medical errors. The IOM Report in 1999, *To Err is Human*,[1] was noted by the media, the public, and political leaders for its startling conclusions, and it initiated the modern patient safety movement.

It has been 16 years since the IOM publication and a patient safety effort has been put into place, particularly for hospitals, in such places as the emergency department, labor and delivery, the intensive care unit (ICU), the operating room

(OR), and anesthesia services. The rate of error remains alarmingly high, however, and some reports using the Institute for Healthcare Improvement (IHI) Global Trigger Tool[2,3] suggest a 10-times higher rate of adverse events than previously estimated. For complex care with seriously ill patients, the risk of error and patient harm is very high (**Box 1**). It is estimated that at least 1 in 10, and as high as 1 in 3, hospital admissions is marred by an adverse event. In the ICU setting, it is expected that there are 1.7 adverse events per day.[4] Unfortunately, unlike the military and the nuclear and aviation industries, medical care has not achieved the status of operation of an HRO in most realms and most communities.

What is patient safety? There can be confusion when discussing patient safety and it is important to distinguish between adverse outcomes as a result of medical care from those that arise from the patient's underlying medical conditions causing morbidity and mortality.[5] As a result of this important difference, an adverse event (or harm) is defined by those outcomes that result from medical care. The IHI defines an adverse surgical event as "any noxious or unintended event occurring in association with medical care to surgical patients."[3] A simpler definition is an injury or harm related to or from the delivery of care. Patients can experience harm as a result of their

---

Box 1
Categories of severity of error

Category A: Circumstances or events that have the capacity to cause error

Category B: An error that did not reach the patient

Category C: An error that reached the patient but did not cause harm

Category D: An error that reached the patient and required monitoring or intervention to confirm that it resulted in no harm to the patient

Category E: Temporary harm to the patient and required intervention

Category F: Temporary harm to the patient and required initial or prolonged hospitalization

Category G: Permanent patient harm

Category H: Intervention required to sustain life

Category I: Patient death

Reprinted with the permission of the National Coordinating Council for Medication Error Reporting and Prevention, ©2001.

medical care in the absence of errors; therefore, adverse events are categorized as preventable and nonpreventable.

Medical error then is defined as an act of commission or omission leading to an undesirable outcome or significant potential for such an outcome.[6] Some errors are harmless, some cause injury, and some are near misses that do not cause injury because they are intercepted by secondary actions or by chance.[7] **Fig. 2** shows the types of errors. There is some debate among experts in defining preventable and nonpreventable events. Some think that events characterized by the Center for Medicare and Medicaid Services as never events cannot always be prevented, whereas others think that labeling nonpreventable events is self-fulfilling and that with better systems these events should be preventable. Negligence occurs when an error occurs below the standard of care and can result in legal liability.

There can be difficulty distinguishing between patient safety and quality of care. Quality of care is defined by the IOM as "the degree to which health services for individuals and populations increase the likelihood of desired health outcomes and are consistent with current professional knowledge."[8] In their less than edifying definition, safety is seen as a subset of a broader umbrella of quality of care. The report lists 6 specific aims for quality improvement in which health care must be: safe, effective, patient-centered, timely, efficient, and equitable. Health care researcher Avedis Donabedian[9] created a methodology of studying quality of care that is currently used extensively and includes how care is organized (structure), what was done (process), and what happened to the patient (outcome). Again, patient safety can be seen emerging in these 3 domains. As a result of efforts to improve both patient safety and patient quality of care, a variety of quality measurements, practice guidelines, and clinical pathways have been developed. These are largely derived from evidence-based medicine and help standardize care. These have helped in many areas but do not allow for individual approaches from expert clinicians and are difficult to use with very complex care with many overlapping illnesses.

The costs of treating patients who suffer from medical error and adverse events are significant and multiple. The IOM estimated that annual costs for preventable and nonpreventable adverse events in the United States in 1999 was between 34 and 58 billion dollars total for lost income, lost household production, disability, and increased health care costs.[1] In addition, there are costs for litigation imposed on society resulting from these occurrences, and there is loss of trust and faith in the health care system and care providers by the public as a result of these events.

Appropriately and importantly, after a medical error or adverse event, the focus should be placed on the patient and the patient family that suffered the error. Patients who have suffered a medical injury require an apology and an explanation of what took place and what will be done to remedy the problem. The emotional impact can be difficult and complex because the unintentional harm is caused by caregivers that the patient had trusted and because those same caregivers often have to provide treatment of the injury.[10] However, the health care provider associated with the error is a second victim in serious adverse events.[11] Health care providers associated with serious adverse events feel embarrassment, guilt, and isolation, and can lose self-confidence, resulting in possible increased risk of future error. The best approach is often a compassionate ear and support from colleagues. Colleagues should avoid judgment and provide support and remind the second victim of how ubiquitous errors are in medicine.[12] Unfortunately, as a result of possible future litigation, health care providers are often advised not to discuss the case with colleagues.

How do patient safety and the practice of oral and maxillofacial surgery intersect? Why would an oral and maxillofacial surgeon (OMS) be concerned about patient safety and how relevant is this topic for an office-based surgeon? Many OMSs have a predominantly office-based practice and only spend a small amount of their typical week in the hospital setting. Most OMSs are familiar with the safety initiatives at their local hospitals and can understand the benefit of such systems. **Box 2** outlines the types of medical errors

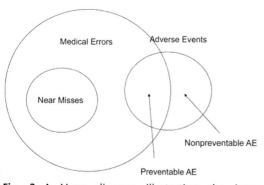

Fig. 2. A Venn diagram illustrating the interrelationships between outcome measures. AE, adverse event. (*From* Camargo CA Jr, Tsai CL, Sullivan AF, et al. Safety climate and medical errors in 62 US emergency departments. Ann Emerg Med 2012;60(5):555–63.e20; with permission.)

Box 2
Types of medical errors affecting oral and maxillofacial surgery patients

Medication errors

- Time frame: Ordering-stage, transcribing-stage, dispensing-stage, administration-stage errors
- Right drug, right route, right dose, right time, right drug
- High-risk abbreviations

Surgical errors

- Wrong site surgery, surgical fires, retained gauze or instruments, health care–associated infections, readmissions

Anesthesia errors

- Failure to recognize patient's physiologic reserve
- Failure of airway assessment,
- Undersedation or oversedation
- Failure to rescue from deeper level of sedation,
- Inadequate preparation and practice for office emergencies

Diagnostic errors

- Failure to diagnose
- Delay in diagnosis
- Misdiagnosis
- Overdiagnosis

Errors of the human–machine interface

- Not understanding how to use diagnostic or therapeutic equipment
- Not understanding limitations of technology

Communication, handoff, and staff errors

- Inadequate or incomplete staff training
- Procedure room to recovery area (OR to post-anesthesia care unit [PACU]), PACU to floor, floor to discharge home
- Staff to staff in office setting
- Doctor to doctor in a multiple doctor office
- Doctor or staff to patient or patient family
- Afterhours coverage of practice or hospital issues

Health care–associated infections

introduces the various types of medical error (see discussion of details, in this issue).

It is estimated that medication errors or adverse drug events (ADEs) occur in 5% of hospitalized patients and an additional 5% to 10% of patients have potential medication errors.[13] In the outpatient setting, a study showed a 1 in 4 rate of ADE over a 3-month period in a large group of outpatients.[14] It is estimated that there are 10,000 prescription drugs and 300,000 over-the-counter products available[15] and, as the population ages, polypharmacy and drug interaction has become a frequent problem for patients and their prescribers. Medicine reconciliation at each transition in the care process has become more important and more critical to minimize error. In emergency carts, particularly, confusion about look-alike, sound-alike drugs can be deadly. The different concentrations of epinephrine (1:1000 vs 1:10,000) and appropriate route are a frequent source of confusion in emergency management courses. Another example of a frequent ADE is the management of anticoagulants. OMSs frequently have to stop and resume anticoagulant medications, which presents a high risk for error and miscommunication.

Surgical errors account for a high proportion of adverse events and traditionally errors were viewed as the fault of a less-than-excellent surgeon. Wrong site and wrong patient surgeries make for jaw dropping headlines in the 24-hour news cycle. Processes, systems, timeouts, and checklists are the structures that allow for reduction of complications (see later discussion). One area of wisdom that has emerged as part of the patient safety movement is the volume–outcomes relationship for both surgeons and hospital systems. Surgeons and hospital systems that have higher volume of procedures tend to have a lower complication rate compared with surgeons and hospital systems that have a lower volume of those procedures.[16,17]

One of the most high profile safety issues in oral and maxillofacial surgery is anesthesia safety. As a specialty, office-based anesthesia has been a core service that OMS are trained for and use well in their surgical office-based practices. The patient safety record has been very good[18,19] but outliers and disasters still occur. Surprisingly, when reviewed, the cases in which anesthesia disasters occur usually involve the same repeated themes of airway assessment, inappropriate patient selection, oversedation, and lack of ability to rescue the patient from a deeper level of sedation than was intended. Modern monitoring, such as pulse oximetry and end-tidal carbon dioxide, have made recognizing impending airway or respiratory

that can occur in treating patients whether in the hospital or office setting. A review of the types of errors reveals that this topic affects all patients and permeates health care treatment. This article compromise much earlier and easier in patient management. Proper airway assessment, excluding patients who are not appropriate candidates for office-based anesthesia, anesthesia depth-limit setting, and emergency management rehearsal and staff training should be part of every oral and maxillofacial surgery office's modus operandi.

With regard to some of the safety issues commonly outlined in studies in the hospital setting (eg, central line–associated bloodstream infection, urinary catheter infection, Clostridium difficile infection, ventilator-associated pneumonia) the office environment is an easier setting in which to manage and implement simplification and standardization of procedures. Patients may be more able to intervene in their safety if they sense that something that is out of the ordinary. The challenge is that, unlike large hospitals with risk managers, compliance officers, medical directors, and quality officers, solo practitioners must manage all these roles essentially on their own. The author has had an office accredited by the Joint Commission for more than 8 years and understands the challenges of even trying to put in place and verify handwashing compliance in the office setting.

Diagnostic errors can arise in several categories such as failure to diagnose, delay in diagnosis, or misdiagnosis. All these categories obviously can cause patient harm. For an OMS, failure to diagnose or delay in diagnosis of premalignant or malignant disease is perhaps the most worrisome. A pathology logbook that is checked weekly and a formal tracking system for patients of concern are needed to prevent patients with suspicious lesions from being lost to follow-up. An area that has not been too much of a concern for an OMS is that of overdiagnosis. The pharmaceutical industry markets heavily to consumers and has caused some to think that overdiagnosis is a problem. Contemporary digital imaging and more specific test results allow visualization and identification of conditions that could not be investigated in the past, resulting in a more frequent rate of diagnosis, which may or may not affect the health of patients.

Errors caused by the human–machine interface have become more commonplace. Although technology and engineering improvements are solutions for some health care problems, understanding the technology and its limitations is imperative as OMSs depend more on modern technology. In the anesthesia realm, a variety of engineering solutions, such as the Pindex system, dissimilar fittings for various gases, failsafe devices, and vaporizer interlocks have made the modern anesthesia machine much safer than earlier counterparts. Challenges remain, however, because modern anesthesia machines have multiple parameter settings and alarm configurations that must be understood and responded to properly. Another example is use of infusion pumps, which can be quite sophisticated. Medication errors related to entering incorrect medication concentration, bolus, and infusion rates must be understood.

One area fraught with difficulty is the broad area of communication between health care providers in different areas of the OMSs practice and in different areas of the hospital. Such information handoffs are critical in tracing a patient's transit through care. The Joint Commission determined that the most frequent elements in root cause analysis (RCA) of a sentinel event (an unexpected serious injury or death) were communication problems, which occurred about 70% of the time (see **Fig. 2**).[20] From the floor to the OR, from the OR to the postanesthesia care unit (PACU), and from PACU to the ICU or step-down unit, there are multiple opportunities for breaches in the continuity of care and multiple opportunities for management and medication error. Similar opportunities for error and harm occur in the office from doctor to doctor, doctor or staff to patient, and doctor to staff during anesthetic cases or, especially, during management of a medical emergency.

Addressing solutions to the problems of patient safety requires a methodology that recognizes that humans are not perfect and that human error occurs in dedicated, well-trained, and hardworking caregivers. It is very difficult to prevent people from making mistakes that they never intended to make and it is not a matter of concentrating harder or acting more carefully. Active error refers to those errors at the delivery of care (the surgeon) versus latent errors that occur away from the bedside, such as low staffing levels that increase the likelihood for error. It is also important to understand that human beings exhibit conscious behavior in which we have to think about a task, and automatic unconscious behaviors in tasks that we have done many times and can do while thinking about other things. Automatic behaviors result in slips, which are a more frequent threat to patient safety because so many tasks are automatic. Conscious behaviors result in mistakes because of lack of knowledge, lack of training, inadequate information, or applying incorrect algorithms to a clinical problem.[5]

An important shift that is gradually taking place with those involved in the patient safety movement but is still largely forthcoming in most health care arenas is away from the blame and shame game to systems thinking. Systems thinking anticipates errors and either prevents the error from penetrating to the patient or intercepts them before they cause harm.[21] In this way, multiple layers of protection exist that shield patients from error by building in redundancies and crosschecks, and creating standardization and simplification. This process can be easier to implement than one might initially think in the office environment. For example, when many OMSs started to perform fixed hybrid cases and immediate denture conversion, a preprocedure, intraprocedure, and postprocedure flowsheet was developed. This flowsheet allowed providers to organize communication (for the team, the patient, and the referring dentist), arrange supplies, and establish timeframes to decrease stress and improve patient outcomes. This type of approach can be applied to more complex care systems. Examples of systems that help reduce the rate of error are listed in **Box 3**. OMSs are still learning how to record, study, and resolve errors and have to recognize hindsight bias. Hindsight bias is the tendency for reviewers of adverse outcomes to see the past event as obvious and stepwise, whereas in real time and real life the decisions that lead to patient harm are not connected in a straight line and information is often insufficient. Another important concept on review of adverse outcomes (within a specialty or hospital system) is the recognition that some patient care activities are at higher risk for error and higher risk for severe outcome than others. Care or treatment tasks that are at high risk for error require more redundancies, standardization, and simplification compared with those at low risk. Blood transfusion protocols are an excellent example of such a task. Charles Vincent and colleagues[22] developed a framework that allows for focus and remediation of the root causes of error. He categorized root causes of errors as belonging to institutional, organizational, work environment, team, individual, task, and patient areas.

A balance between systems thinking and just culture versus accountability must be developed to develop a culture of safety. Previous discussion focused on systems thinking to limit exposure and penetration of error to patients and on how to protect health care providers from being prone to error. There are disruptive behaviors and reckless behaviors that do exist and must be addressed; therefore, lines must be drawn between acceptable and unacceptable behavior. What should be done when a staff member repeatedly makes the same mistakes and does not improve competency? What should be done when an individual knowingly engages in an unsafe act? Leonard and Frankel[23] developed an algorithm that asks 3 questions that lead to a decision whether or not discipline of the care provider is warranted. First, it asks whether the caregiver's thinking was impaired, malicious, risky, or unintentional. Second, it asks if other caregivers with the same training and experience would make the same mistake. Finally, it asks if the care provider has a history of unsafe acts. This review process is conducted independently of whether or not patient harm occurred.

Staff training and staff competency are very important for patient safety. The Joint Commission advocates that "good care starts with good staff."[24] It seems instinctive that a well-trained, well-staffed, and well-rested workforce is important in delivering safe care. In the nursing realm, data exist to show that increased patient load, longer work hours, and high patient turnover leads to poorer outcomes and higher rate of medical errors.[25,26] Although counterintuitive, there are little data linking patient safety to the work hours of a practicing physician. After 3 decades as an OMS, the author can state anecdotally that the ability to function and make decisions well after little sleep the night before is hampered compared with a well-rested state. When feeling poorly, after vacation, or when the normal routine at the office has been disrupted for whatever reason (construction, new equipment, change in personnel, new techniques), a more scripted, methodical approach using templates is likely to improve patient safety.

Box 3
Examples of systems to enhance patient safety

- Surgical timeout (correct patient, correct site, correct procedure, imaging marked correctly, implants and devices available, correct documentation)
- Using 2 patient identifiers
- Read back procedure for verbal orders
- Identifying look-alike, sound-alike drugs and separating them
- Medicine reconciliation
- Removal of life-threatening drugs from floors to the pharmacies
- Anesthesia machine checklist
- Emergency cart checklist
- Pathology logbook
- Blood transfusion protocols
- Regular emergency drills in office
- Electronic prescription writing

For oral and maxillofacial surgery with the anesthesia team delivery model, staff training for the office anesthesia assistant is a key element in patient safety. Staff training for airway management, preparation for office emergencies, and understanding of the variety of sedation and general anesthetic techniques, as well as recovery and discharge criteria, helps minimize risk in patient management. More than 20 years' experience in private practice leads the author to conclude that staff training takes more time to complete and more follow-up than might be imagined to ensure that staff really have the understanding of a new technique, new equipment, and so forth. Competency training for staff is an ongoing and career-long process, and is a moving target.

Closely aligned with staff training and staff competency are crew resource management (CRM) and teamwork training in health care. CRM grew out of the aviation industry in the late 1970s and early 1980s after some landmark accidents caused the National Aeronautics and Space Administration and the aviation industry to examine procedures, communication, hierarchy of command, management of information, situational awareness, and teamwork to address safety concerns (**Box 4**). Although many analogies to the aviation industry exist, health care is different in that health care often involves more complex tasks, is less automated, and decision-making in the face of incomplete information is less linear. However, much can be learned in team training exercises. Team training exercises focus on improving communication skills, creating a more cohesive environment, and leveling the hierarchy of command so all providers can give input and speak up without fear of reprimand, allowing for use of briefs and debriefs on critical events.[27,28] Other key elements of team training include allocation of resources, the use of cognitive aids, and use of all available information and help in critical situations. The literature has been slow to show benefit of team training on outcomes but some studies are strongly supportive.[29]

Simulation training has become an important part of medical education and enhancing patient safety. Simulation training offers a unique learning experience that allows for input from other high-risk industries in task analysis and then incorporates concepts of CRM, stress inoculation training, deliberate practice, and interprofessional team training, as well as reduces patient risk. Simulation allows for consistent training and assessment. Simulation training offers risk-free skill rehearsal, assessment, and feedback. Simulation training has been shown to be effective in knowledge transfer, is well proven in certain technical skills teaching, and is less well proven in nontechnical skills training. Generalization of the effectiveness of simulation training to improved clinical care is still relatively absent and it is unclear if effectiveness in a scenario transfers to another scenario[30–33] (**Box 5**). Simulation training seems to be the best way to prepare for rare but potentially life-threatening emergencies. The American Association of Oral and Maxillofacial Surgeons has made a substantial investment in simulation training as it relates to anesthesia management of airway challenges and emergency management to enhance patient safety.

SAFETY CULTURE

At the beginning of this article, operations on an aircraft carrier deck, the inherent risk, and the safety record were discussed. An HRO is an organization that carries out tasks with a high potential for error but has few adverse outcomes. A goal for a health care organization is to strive to be an HRO. The characteristics of an HRO are summarized in **Box 6**.[34] A safety culture promotes trust and empowers staff to report errors, near misses, and risks.[35] Importantly, accountability is a key factor in safety culture. Staff must be comfortable admitting their own mistakes and also monitoring

---

Box 4
Crew resource management

Situational awareness (maintain and recover)

Communication (efficiency, overcoming barriers)

Task management (using cognitive aids, delegation)

Coordination (teamwork)

Decision-making (problem-solving)

Care or treatment planning (before, during, after)

Box 5
Simulation training

- Provides active and experiential learning
- Familiarization with equipment and medications
- Deliberate and reflective practice of rare events
- Organize and optimize operations
- Encourage use of checklists and cognitive aids
- Practice CRM
- Share best practices

Box 6
Characteristics of a high-reliability organization

- Preoccupation with failure (being aware of error and potential for error)
- Reluctance to simplify (understanding complexity of work)
- Sensitivity to operations (awareness of front-line work)
- Deference to expertise (allow frontline workers to make decisions)
- Commitment to resilience (identify, contain, and improve from error)

the work of those around them. Finally, improvement must take place and it must be communicated to the staff that their concerns have been addressed. As previously discussed, creating, and maintaining a just culture is a core element to enable staff to admit their mistakes.

Despite efforts at reducing error, errors will still occur and evaluating how and why an event occurred is part of an RCA analysis. The elements in RCA are outlined in **Box 7**.[36] Ultimately, the purpose of the RCA is to reduce or eliminate the causes of the error to reduce risk of patient harm. Once the causes are determined, a variety of actions can take place to change processes, make physical changes, improve workload, use checklists, create policies, or implement training to address the causes. Finally, transparency may be the important final step so that the system can be adapted and improved.[37]

John Powell[38] said "the only real mistake is the one from which we learn nothing." Patient care is a complex process that has high risk for error

Box 7
Root cause analysis review of factors that lead to latent error

- Institutional or regulatory
- Organizational or management
- Work environment
- Team environment
- Staffing
- Task-related
- Patient characteristics

Adapted with permission from AHRQ Patient Safety Network: Ranji S, Wachter RM, Hartman EE. Patient Safety Primer: Root Cause Analysis. AHRQ Patient Safety Network. Available at: https://psnet.ahrq.gov/primers/primer/10. Updated July 2016.

and it is critical that OMSs learn from their mistakes to improve patient safety and improve care outcomes. Whether managing patients in private offices or as part of a care team at hospitals, OMSs owe it to patients to understand medical error and take action to reduce its frequency and adverse effects. This article reviewed general concepts of patient safety and the reader is encouraged to further explore this topic.

Resources in Patient Safety

Book:
 Understanding Patient Safety by Robert Wachter, MD. This excellent book is a quick read and great overview of the current status and challenges of the patient safety movement.

Web resources:
 Agency for Healthcare Research and Quality (http://ahrq.gov?) is a federal program to make health care safer and with higher quality. It has many resources for the public and health care workers.
 Anesthesia Patient Safety Foundation (http://apsf.org) is an organization to continually improve the safety of patients undergoing anesthesia.
 Institute for Healthcare Improvement (http://ihi.org) is an organization to improve health care worldwide.
 Joint Commission (http://jointcommission.org) is an independent nonprofit organization that has a lot of information related to health care and patient safety. It tends to be a bureaucratic organization that is rigid but has good resources.
 Leapfrog Group (http://leapfroggroup.org) is a coalition with the goal of improving quality and safety in hospital systems.
 Institute for Safe Medication Practices (http://ismp.org) is an organization devoted to medication error and safe medication use.
 OMSNIC (http://dds4dds.com) is a risk management company for oral and maxillofacial surgery, they have very good Web resources and good seminars that provide education and reduce patient risk for adverse events.

REFERENCES

1. Kohn L, Corrigan J, Donaldson M, editors. To err is human; building a safer health system. Washington, DC: Committee on Quality of Health Care in America, Institute of Medicine: National Academy Press; 2000.

2. Classen DC, Resar R, Griffin F, et al. "Global Trigger Tool" shows that adverse events in hospitals may be ten times greater than previously measured. Health Aff 2011;30(4):581–9.

3. Available at: http://www.ihi.org/resources/Pages/IHIWhitePapers/IHIGlobalTriggerToolWhitePaper.aspx. Accessed February 6, 2016.

4. Donchin Y, Gopher D, Olin M, et al. A look into the nature and causes of human errors in the intensive care unit. Crit Care Med 1995;23:294–300.

5. Wachter R. Understanding patient safety. 2nd edition. New York: McGraw Hill Medical; 2012.

6. Available at: www.webmm.ahrq.gov/glossary.aspx. Accessed February 7, 2016.

7. Available at: www.psnet.ahrq.gov/primers. Accessed February 7, 2016.

8. Committee on Quality of Health Care in America, Institute of Medicine. Crossing the quality chasm: a new health system for the 21st century. Washington, DC: National Academy Press; 2001.

9. Donabedian A. The quality of care. How can it be assessed? JAMA 1988;260:1743–8.

10. Vincent C. Patient safety. 2nd edition. West Sussex (United Kingdom): Wiley-Blackwell; 2010.

11. Wu AW. Medical error: the second victim. BMJ 2000;320:726–7.

12. Hershey K. Culture of safety. Nurs Clin North Am 2015;50:139–52.

13. Bates DW, Cullen DJ, Laird N, et al. Incidence of adverse drug events and potential adverse drug events. Implications for prevention. ADE Prevention Study Group. JAMA 1995;274:29–34.

14. Gandhi TK, Weingart SN, Borus J, et al. Adverse drug events in ambulatory care. N Engl J Med 2003;348:1556–64.

15. Aspden P, Wolcott J, Bootman JL, et al, editors. Committee on Identifying and Preventing Medication Errors. Preventing medication errors: quality chasm series. Institute of Medicine. Washington, DC: The National Academy Press; 2007.

16. Eggli Y, Halfon P, Meylan D, et al. Surgical safety and hospital volume across a wide range of interventions. Med Care 2010;48:962–71.

17. Luft HS, Bunker JP, Enthoven AC. Should operations be regionalized? The empirical relation between surgical volume and mortality. N Engl J Med 1979;301:1364–9.

18. D'Eramo E, Bookless S, Howard J. Adverse events in outpatient anesthesia in Massachusetts. JOMS 2003;61(7):793–800.

19. Other article on OMS safety.

20. Available at: http://www.jointcommission.org/assets/1/18/Root_Causes_by_Event_Type_2004-2015.pdf. Accessed March 5, 2016.

21. Reason JT. Managing the risks of organizational accidents. Aldershots (United Kingdom): Ashgate; 1997.

22. Vincent C, Talor-Adams S, Stanhorpe N. Understanding and responding to adverse events. N Engl J Med 2003;348:1051–6.

23. Leonard MW, Frankel A. The path to safe and reliable healthcare. Patient Educ Couns 2010;80:288–92.

24. Available at: http://www.centerfortransforminghealthcare.org/about_us.aspx. Accessed July 16, 2016.

25. Aieken LH, Clarke SP, Sloane DM, et al. Hospital nurse staffing and patient mortality, nurse burnout, and job dissatisfaction. JAMA 2002;288:1987–93.

26. Needleman J, Buerhaus P, Pankratz VS, et al. Nurse staffing and inpatient hospital mortality. N Engl J Med 2011;364:1037–45.

27. Maynard MT, Marshall D, Dean MD. Crew Resource Management and Teamwork Training in Health Care: A Review of the literature and recommendations for how to leverage such interventions to enhance patient safety. Annual Review of Health Care Management: Strategy and Policy Perspectives on Reforming Health Systems. Adv Health Care Manag 2012;13:59–91.

28. Frankel A. Patient safety: anesthesia in remote locations. Anesthesiol Clin 2009;27:127–39.

29. Neily J, Mills PD, Young-Xu Y, et al. Association between implementation of a medical team training program and surgical mortality. JAMA 2010;304:1693–700.

30. Cook DA, Erwin PJ, Triola MM. Computerized virtual patients in health professions education: a systematic review and meta analysis. Acad Med 2010;85:1589–602.

31. Cook DA, Hatala R, Brydges R, et al. Technology-enhanced simulation for health professions education: a systematic review and meta-analysis. JAMA 2011;306:978–88.

32. Zendejas B, Brydges R, Wang AT, et al. Patient outcomes in simulation-based medical education: a systematic review. J Gen Intern Med 2013;28(8):1078–89.

33. Croskerry P. Cognitive forcing strategies in clinical decision making. Ann Emerg Med 2003;41(1):110–20.

34. Chassin MR, Loeb JM. High-reliability health care: getting there from here. Milbank Q 2013;91:459–90.

35. Croskerry P. Universal model of diagnostic reasoning. Acad Med 2009;84(8):1022–88.

36. Available at: https://psnet.ahrq.gov/primers/primer/10/root-cause-analysis. Accessed May 20, 2016.

37. Weick KE, Sutcliffe KM. Managing the unexpected: assuring high performance in an age of complexity. San Francisco (CA): Jossey-Bass; 2001.

38. Powell J. The Secret of Staying in Love. Tabor Pulbishing, Pennsylvainia State University; 1990.

Preoperative Preparation and Planning of the Oral and Maxillofacial Surgery Patient

Jeffrey D. Bennett, DMD

KEYWORDS

- Patient preparation • Medical history • Medication reconciliation • Airway assessment
- Postoperative analgesia • Postoperative nausea and vomiting • Perioperative antibiotics
- Transference of care

KEY POINTS

- Understanding who the patient is requires obtaining a complete and accurate medical history.
- Not all patients are the same – caring for the pediatric, geriatric, and medically compromised patient present different concerns.
- Systems should be implemented to alert the office and practitioner to critical aspects of patient care, which can minimize errors.
- One size fits all is inappropriate in regard to postoperative analgesia.
- Routine postoperative antibiotics are usually not indicated.
- Optimizing patient outcome requires a plan for transference of care when the primary surgeon is not available.

INTRODUCTION

Ensuring patient safety depends on many variables. Each, when not fully addressed, increases the potential for patient harm. This article focuses on patient preparation. The goal of patient preparation is to ensure that the patient is in optimal condition to proceed with the planned procedure. This requires that the surgeon know who the patient is by obtaining a complete and accurate medical history, including medication reconciliation and tracking the results of all laboratory, diagnostic, and imaging studies. Patient optimization ensures that the surgeon strives for the best results; recognizes perioperative risks, which can contribute to an adverse event are identified and managed; minimizes and controls perioperative pain; is judicious in case selection; and arranges continuance of care throughout the perioperative period.

MEDICAL HISTORY

The first step in patient preparation is to obtain a complete medical history. Without such, the practitioner does not truly know their patient. Accreditation standards for predoctoral dental education dictate that a student is competent in obtaining a medical history. Many before me have written about the application of this standard, and the difference in opinion of many educators as to its satisfactory achievement with some feeling that there is a significant disregard for patient medical assessment in dental education, minimizing the accreditation standard.[1–3] Understanding the

Disclosure: This article has no commercial or financial conflicts of interest and has received no support from external funding sources.
1481 West 10th Street, Indianapolis, IN 46202, USA
E-mail address: jb2omfs@gmail.com

Oral Maxillofacial Surg Clin N Am 29 (2017) 131–140
http://dx.doi.org/10.1016/j.coms.2016.12.005
1042-3699/17/© 2017 Elsevier Inc. All rights reserved.

importance of the medical history and physical examination, oral and maxillofacial surgery accreditation standards require a distinct course in medical history taking and physical examination for all residents.

The medical history provides information about the patient's past and present history and consists of past medical history, past surgical history, social history, medications, allergies, and a review of systems. Each component is critical. Any incomplete or contradictory information between sections must be explained, investigated, and/or clarified. Filling the informational gaps may be as straightforward as identifying a justification as to why the patient is taking a specific medication (eg, clarifying why a patient is taking an antihypertensive medication when the patient does not list a history of hypertension) or inquiring as to whether the patient is, has stopped, or should be on a medication for a specific condition identified in the medical history (eg, clarifying why a patient with a history of atrial fibrillation is not taking an anticoagulant).

Medical intake forms are usually good for providing a checklist of medical conditions (eg, hypertension) for the practitioner and/or patient to check off. A prepared checklist provides a foundation from which a medical intake can begin. For the individual with low health literacy, however, the form may be confusing and the individual may incorrectly respond "no" to many of the questions. Many patients may not have seen a physician for several years and the medical history responses reflecting a negative health history may not reveal the patient's actual health. A prepared checklist is also usually insufficient in allowing full documentation of a review of systems. The review of systems would detail the severity of a known disease or identify potentially undiagnosed disorders, clarifying potential inconsistencies in a checklist medical history form.

Fortunately, for most practitioners a significant percentage of their patients are young and healthy, and a review of systems is noncontributory and can be completed quickly. However, for the geriatric patient, the medically compromised patient, or the patient with an unrecognized condition, the review of systems may entail a detailed discussion and provide significant information that may alter the planned treatment.

Accepting a patient-completed unremarkable health form, using an abbreviated medical history without obtaining a review of system despite understanding the inadequacy and potential for missed information is the act of neglecting or doing something wrong, which is an "act of commission." Failing to understand the necessity or lack of knowledge to obtain a complete review of systems is a failure to do the correct thing, which is an "act of omission."[4] This failure does not necessarily result in an undesirable outcome. At times, a significant adverse event may occur that is successfully managed by the primary team without any long-term sequelae. The lack of an adverse event, the lack of recognizing an adverse event, or the management of a "close call" may actually contribute to the sense by the practitioner that their abbreviated history taking methodology is sufficient, regardless of whether they appreciate the deficiency in the history and the missing information.

MEDICATION RECONCILIATION

Many patients who present to the oral and maxillofacial surgeon are taking multiple prescribed and over-the-counter medications. This is most prevalent in the geriatric population, where approximately 36% of the patients are taking 5 or more medications weekly.[5] Herbal or dietary supplements may not routinely be inquired about when taking a medical history, yet up to approximately 20% of the population may be taking such a supplement with an even higher percentage of use among the elderly population, with 1 study reporting approximately two-thirds of the elderly population using one such supplement.[5–7]

Medication reconciliation is a critical safety matter. It is the process by which the practitioner establishes a complete and accurate a list of medications that the patient is taking. The process in which to gather this information may be challenging and time consuming, because many patients may neither accurately maintain a record of what they are prescribed nor what they are taking. Asking the patient to bring their medication bottles with them to the appointment, inquiring from family, requesting the information from the patient's primary care doctor, or contacting the pharmacy are potential sources of information. When a patient receives care from multiple physicians, each of these doctors may be prescribing medications. The oral and maxillofacial surgeon cannot assume that each of these doctors has been in contact with the patient's other doctors and thus they have a complete and accurate list of medications. With more than 1 doctor prescribing medications, if communication between doctors is lacking there may be a higher likelihood of a potential drug–drug interaction, which may be unrecognized and not manifest itself until surgery or medications prescribed by the oral and maxillofacial surgeon. With advancements in information technology and the electronic medical record, the process to reconcile medications will improve. As arduous as it currently may be, it is the practitioner's responsibility to obtain medication reconciliation.

It is critical that the oral and maxillofacial surgeon know what medications the patient is taking. This is critical for both planning and implementing treatment. Adverse drug interactions may occur throughout the perioperative period. Preoperatively, a patient may not modify their diabetic medication resulting in a hypoglycemic event. This may occur in the sedated patient specifically directed to be NPO or any diabetic patient who alters their normal routine in anticipation of the planned procedure. Epinephrine in the local anesthetic can interact with nonselective beta-blockers. Antipsychotic and neurologic medications can potentiate the effects of anesthetic agents. Chronic antihypertensive medications may result in a greater possibility of hypotension refractory to treatment or hypertension, depending on whether the medication was continued or discontinued before the surgery and anesthetic. Antiplatelet and anticoagulant medications may increase bleeding in the surgical field. Although there may remain some controversy as to how to manage patients on antiplatelet and anticoagulant medications, most surgeons would agree that most of the time for dentoalveolar procedures, including extraction of impacted third molars and excision of mandibular tori, these medications (including the newer direct thrombin and factor Xa inhibitors) can be continued.[8–10] The medication is continued (with appropriate monitoring of laboratory tests for selected medications), because the risk of an embolic event with discontinuance of the medication, is unnecessary, because local hemostatic measures usually control any surgery-associated bleeding.

Errors may be the result of unconscious behavior. There are many tasks that the surgeon does automatically, repeated several times a day, usually without adverse consequence. The more distracting the environment the more likely that this unconscious behavior can contribute to an adverse outcome. Adverse drug interactions may occur as a result of a postoperative medication prescribed by the oral and maxillofacial surgeon. Antibiotics may alter gut flora causing pseudomembranous colitis, or alter drug availability, absorption and/or metabolization, for example, resulting in an increase in the international normalized ratio in a patient prescribed warfarin.

Adverse drug effects may also occur during the postoperative period secondary to not monitoring the use of chronic medications. Surgery alters dietary intake, and anesthesia and postoperative analgesia have emetic potential, both of which can contribute to a hypoglycemic event in the postoperative period if appropriate instructions and interventions are not provided to the diabetic patient. Last, it is critical that an adequate amount of time is provided with the patient and their family to ensure that they fully understand and verify an understanding of the oral/written instructions regarding all postoperative medications.

TRACKING DATA

A patient's care can traverse many offices. Examples of this may include the interaction between the oral and maxillofacial surgeon with the primary care provider or pharmacy, to clarify a medical history or reconcile a patient's medications, respectively. This encounter usually precedes treatment. The surgeon may also order laboratory tests, diagnostic studies, imaging studies, or submit pathologic specimens for diagnosis. Tracking of these studies and ensuring patient follow-up is also critical to patient care.[11] Failure to track data is a system error and was identified as the root cause for missed, delayed, or erroneous diagnoses in approximately 70% of cases identified through quality assurance.[12]

A clearly defined and developed system can be established at several levels. The office is responsible for (1) a specimen obtained in the office is appropriately transported and received at the diagnostic facility; (2) ensuring that the patient follows through with a laboratory test, or diagnostic or imaging study that has been ordered and is to be obtained in a different facility; (3) ensuring that the ordered test/study results are received, reviewed, and consistent with the patient's differential diagnosis; (4) partnering with a laboratory or diagnostic facility that ensures that all abnormal results are communicated with the office; (5) scheduling a follow-up appointment for any test or study ordered that also establishes an alert if this appointment is canceled or missed. The ordering practitioner must also review all tests and studies.

Patients may also get involved with their care. This entails the office educating the patient as to the importance of the test or study. Patients who have not received information about a test or study after a specified time (that is not excessive) should contact the office to discuss the results. Some offices may provide the patient with access to their medical records, which could flag any abnormal result alerting the patient to follow up with the practitioner if the office has not yet contacted them.

Today's technology with the cooperative effort of the office, practitioner, and patient has the ability to establish a near fail-safe system. However, no system is fail-safe if the office does not establish a culture of patient safety understanding the complexity of a busy office and the persistent risk that exists for errors to occur.

AIRWAY ASSESSMENT

Adverse respiratory events were the primary factor contributing to morbidity and mortality as identified by the American Society of Anesthesiologists (ASA) closed claims cases published in the late 1980s and early 1990s.[13] A 2009 manuscript that focused on anesthesia delivery in "remote locations" found similar results, with approximately 50% of the cases associated with monitored anesthesia care.[14] Drs Dembo and Bennett also found adverse respiratory events to account for the highest percentage of morbidity and mortality for ambulatory office-based anesthetics identified from American Association of Oral and Maxillofacial Surgeons National closed claims data for the 10-year period between 1989 and 1998. Although the highest incidence of adverse events was respiratory in nature, there was no information that concluded an inadequate airway assessment was contributory to the adverse event. Regardless, prevention of an adverse respiratory event entails a preoperative airway history and examination, and diligent perioperative airway monitoring. The latter will be discussed elsewhere in this issue.

The airway history should identify disease processes that can compromise airway integrity and/or impact airway management (**Box 1**). The examination should identify physical features that in the sedated patient may increase airway collapsibility or obstruction, make airway ventilation difficult or impossible, and/or make intubation difficult or impossible. Although there are criteria that assess difficulty of both mask ventilation (**Box 2**) and intubation (**Box 3**), there are limitations with the sensitivity, specificity, positive predictive value, and negative predictive value of these tools. Because airway management in deep sedation or general anesthesia is unique in which the surgical site infringes on the airway and does not allow simultaneous airway control, there is no specific list of features scientifically validated to identify an increase in airway obstruction and difficulty with airway management.

The physical examination of the airway should minimally include maximal interincisal opening (3 finger breaths), thyromental distance (3 finger breaths), distance between the thyroid cartilage and hyoid bone (2 finger breaths), the Mallampatti-Samsoon classification, neck flexion and extension, and tonsillar hypertrophy. A record

that provides documentation of these specific features of the physical examination is advantageous.

PREEMPTIVE MANAGEMENT OF NAUSEA AND VOMITING

Anesthetic and postoperative agents including nitrous oxide, ketamine, and opioids, as well as surgical consequences, such as swallowed blood, can contribute to postoperative nausea and vomiting. For the patient, besides being distressing it

---

Box 1
Medical disease with potential impact on airway integrity and management

Asthma

Obesity

Snoring

Obstructive sleep apnea

Muscular dystrophy

Myasthenia gravis

Burn patients

Radiation therapy

Poorly controlled diabetes

Rheumatoid arthritis

Down syndrome

Spinal cord injuries

Past head and neck surgery (eg, pharyngeal flap)

Past airway surgery

Box 2
Features associated with potential difficulty with intubation

Maximal interincisive distance

Thyromental distance

Thyrohyoid distance

Mallampatti–Samsoon classification

Position of larynx

Short neck

Neck circumference

Neck hyperextension

Obesity

Facial burns

Lingual tonsil hypertrophy

Skeletal abnormalities

Box 3
Features associated with potential difficulty in mask ventilation

Facial hair

BMI greater than 26 kg/m^2

Edentulousness

Age greater than 55 years

History of snoring

can contribute to wound dehiscence, esophageal injury, dehydration, and electrolyte abnormalities. Early onset of postoperative nausea and vomiting can delay office discharge. In a patient with diabetes, the inability to take in appropriate glucose can potentially result in hypoglycemia with its associated morbidity and mortality.

The incidence of postoperative nausea and vomiting associated with ambulatory oral and maxillofacial surgery has not been investigated extensively; but has been reported to be as high as 20%.[15] Risk factors that increase the incidence of postoperative nausea and vomiting include female sex, younger age, anesthetic agents and postoperative opioids, and a history of postoperative nausea and vomiting or motion sickness. Factors that are conflicting as to whether they increase the risk of postoperative nausea and vomiting include ASA physical status and menstrual cycle.

Propofol has significant antiemetic properties. It is not as well-known that as little as 2 mg of midazolam administered 30 minutes before the end of surgery has antiemetic effects. Decadron 4 mg intravenous, which is administered by many surgeons for its antiinflammatory properties to decrease postoperative swelling, also has antiemetic properties that the literature has reported to be as efficacious as ondansetron 4 mg intravenous. Lastly, rehydrating the patient who presents NPO with a fluid deficit that may exceed 1 L has been shown to make the patient feel better and possibly reduce the risk of postoperative nausea and vomiting.

These concepts are frequently a routine component of the anesthetic regardless of whether the patient is at risk for postoperative nausea and vomiting. For the patient who is considered at high risk for postoperative nausea and vomiting, the surgeon may consider these additional strategies: avoid emetic anesthetic agents, minimize perioperative opioids, scheduled postoperative nonsteroidal analgesics, and combination antiemetic therapy using 2 agents

from 2 different pharmacologic classes. An effective combination would be to prophylactically administer ondansetron, which is a serotonin receptor antagonist, in combination with decadron. If the patient has emesis despite the prophylactic antiemetic administration, the administration of an alternative antiemetic agent may be considered.

There are a number of different classes of agents that are available and can be administered. Complications may include extrapyramidal effects associated with agents that act on the dopamine receptor; neuroleptic malignant syndrome, which is a life-threatening neurologic disorder that may be induced by drugs, such as metoclopramide; and QT prolongation, which "black boxed" droperidol despite not occurring with the low dosage used as an antiemetic, which may be associated with agents such as antihistamines and selective receptor antagonists (eg, ondansetron).

PROPHYLACTIC ANTIBIOTICS

Surgical intervention violates the integrity of an intact membrane and as such there is a concern with microbial contamination and the risk for postoperative infection. Intraoral procedures, including exodontia, implants, intraoral bone grafts, and orthognathic surgery, are classified as clean-contaminated wounds. An open wound, such as sustained from a traumatic injury that communicates through the mucosa/skin (eg, compound mandible fracture) is classified as a contaminated wound.

Prophylactic antibiotic administration is defined as the administration of antibiotics before a procedure in which microbial contamination will occur with the intent to prevent infection. A meta-analyses analyzing data from 250 clinical trials was published in 2009 supported the concept of prophylactic antibiotics.[16] Antibiotic use is not without risk, which may include an adverse reaction, delayed onset of an infection, development of antibiotic resistance, and antibiotic-associated colitis. Antibiotic prophylaxis entails administering the antibiotic appropriate for the potential microbial contamination before the surgical insult at a high enough dosage to establish an appropriate bacteriologic titer. If the surgery extends beyond the half-life of the antibiotic, the antibiotic can be redosed. There is a limited quantity of scientifically valid literature that assesses the perioperative use of antibiotics for various oral and maxillofacial surgery procedures. The literature does tend to support that the administration of a single dose of preoperative antibiotic reduces the incidence of infection for partial and full bony impacted third molar surgery, major surgery such as fracture reduction and orthognathic surgery, and reduces implant and bone graft failure.[17–19] The trials involving third molar surgery are limited and the quality of evidence to dictate that prophylactic antibiotics are mandated is not absolute. Antibiotic prophylaxis (if not used routinely) may be considered based on clinical judgment in patients with increased risk such as those with comorbid medical conditions and in older patients. Antibiotic administration beyond the perioperative period is not supported and can increase the risk of harm to the patient.[20] There is no scientific basis for the administration of postoperative antibiotics without the administration of a preoperative dose unless an intraoperative finding dictates such.

PREOPERATIVE, INTRAOPERATIVE, AND POSTOPERATIVE PAIN CONTROL

It is the surgeon's responsibility to manage the acute pain associated with surgery. There are various options that are available. Understanding the options allows the surgeon to develop a plan that is appropriate for the patient and the proposed surgery.

Postoperative medications frequently prescribed include the peripherally and centrally acting classes of medications: nonsteroidal antiinflammatory drugs (NSAIDs), aspirin, acetaminophen, and opioids. Surgical trauma results in release of peripheral inflammatory and algesic mediators. NSAIDs have an advantage over acetaminophen and opioids in that they are potent inhibitors of the local inflammatory response. NSAIDs have been demonstrated to provide better analgesia than acetaminophen, aspirin, and a single-entity opioid and as effective analgesia as combinations containing opioids with acetaminophen.[21,22] Ibuprofen, an over-the-counter NSAID formulation, provides maximal analgesia at 400 mg with a relatively low risk compared with other NSAIDS for gastrointestinal toxicity.[23,24] The preemptive administration of an NSAID shortly before surgery or immediately afterward, before the waning of the effect of the local anesthetic, and continued at a fixed schedule for the first 48 hours has demonstrated a reduction in the severity of acute surgical pain.[25] NSAIDs compared with opioids have a lower incidence of nausea and vomiting, and sedation.[26]

An additional consideration to attenuate postoperative pain is the administration of a long-acting local anesthetic. Bupivicaine 0.5% with epinephrine 1:200,000 compared with lidocaine 2% with epinephrine 1:100,000 administered as

an inferior alveolar nerve block provided more profound pain relief during the initial short-term anesthetic effect of the bupivacaine, which then persisted for the first 48 hours.[27] Liposomal bupivacaine, which is administered as an infiltrate to the buccal region of the third molar provides efficacious pain reduction for up to 72 hours without the associated prolonged mentolabial anesthesia associated with an inferior alveolar nerve block.

Despite the evidence demonstrating that NSAIDs provide comparable if not superior analgesia than opioid/acetaminophen combinations with fewer adverse side effects, why are opioids or opioid/acetaminophen drugs the most prescribed class of analgesic? The concern is not solely with the specific drug, but also with the quantity prescribed. There may be numerous contributing factors, including patient expectation, patient satisfaction, what the other doctors in the referring area are doing, an inability to call in a refill because hydrocodone was reclassified from a schedule 3 to a schedule 2 drug, and a desire not to be disturbed after hours.[28] There is an opioid epidemic in the United States, which is resulting partially from the diversion of legitimate prescriptions.[29–32] The challenge is to prescribe just the "right" amount; ideally never underprescribing, but routinely prescribing an excessive amount to all patients, for the few who may legitimately require such contributes to the problem.

The surgeon must have the ability to prescribe the necessary analgesia appropriate for the patient and the completed surgery. However, it is important to make those decisions based on evidence and recognize the epidemic that we are facing. Sometimes, changing habits and educating patients may provide comparable if not better results with fewer side effects and without the negative consequences that a practitioner may fear.

PATIENT POPULATIONS
The Pediatric Patient

An ongoing debate exists as to what age range defines the pediatric patient. The American Academy of Pediatrics defines the child as 2 to 12 years of age and the adolescent as 12 to 21 years of age. Oral and maxillofacial surgery defines the pediatric patient as younger then 18 years of age as it pertains to accreditation standards regarding anesthetic care.

Why are we concerned with age? There are behavioral, anatomic, and physiologic differences that impact patient care. A significant component of oral and maxillofacial surgery practice consists of office-based anesthesia. As such, our focus on the pediatric patient concentrates on the anatomic and physiologic maturation, which impact anesthetic care. The child is more susceptible to upper airway obstruction secondary to hypertrophy of the adenoids and tonsils, a large tongue that is positioned higher in the oral cavity impinging on the soft palate, and a compliant trachea. The child has less ability to overcome upper airway obstruction secondary to thoracic muscular fatigue and rib angulation. The child has less functional reserve secondary to decreased alveoli and increased metabolic demand. If the child's airway becomes obstructed or their respirations decrease secondary to anesthetic medication, they desaturate more than twice as rapidly as an adult. The cardiovascular system is also not developed fully in the child. There are physiologic differences, which can manifest themselves if not careful. The child has a less compliant myocardium and increased parasympathetic tone increasing the susceptibility to hypotension that is rate dependent. Significant maturation in the pediatric anatomy and physiology occur between 8 and 12 years of age that minimize the differences between the pediatric and adult patient, decreasing the potential for the occurrence of adverse events.

The Geriatric Patient

It is more difficult to define what is old age. Chronologically, it is defined as age 65 years and beyond. There is a functional decline in physiologic functions (which is differentiated from pathologic changes) with aging that impact all organ systems. As we age, we have less reserve when subjected to physiologic stresses. There is, however, a large variability between patients; although the physiologic changes occur in all individuals, they may not occur at the same rate. There are patients who are old at 50 and those who are young at 80. Changes in the respiratory system all contribute to a decreased efficiency in respiratory function. Respiratory changes associated with aging include (1) less efficacious airway dilator musculature contributing to airway obstruction, (2) cervical arthritis limiting neck extension potentially compromising airway opening, (3) diminished laryngeal reflexes and depressed lower esophageal sphincter tone impairing protection against aspiration, and (4) decreased resting Pao_2, and decreased response to hypoxia and hypercarbia resulting in an increased incidence of oxygen desaturation and apnea. Physiologic and anatomic changes also occur in the cardiovascular system with aging. Some of these are autonomic dysfunction and decreased distensibility of the vascular system, which can result in dysrhthymias (eg, bradycardia), hypotension, and increased myocardial work. Although there is a differentiation between physiologic and pathologic changes with aging, age is also associated with an increased incidence of cardiovascular pathology, such as coronary artery disease.

Anesthetic Management: The Risk

There are millions of anesthetics performed in the oral and maxillofacial surgeon's office annually. Most of these proceed without complications. However, there are rare instances of adverse outcomes. Estimates from the OMS National Insurance Company (OMSNIC) are there is an occurrence of 1 patient death or brain injury per every 348,602 anesthetic procedures.[33] The OMSNIC data do not demonstrate an increased incidence of morbidity or mortality based on age or ASA status. Additionally, neither the data from OMSNIC nor any other databank assesses modifications in anesthetic management in the oral and maxillofacial surgeons office based on age. However, the anatomic and physiologic differences in the pediatric and geriatric patient, as well as the differences in the pharmacodynamic and pharmacokinetic actions of the anesthetic agents intuitively suggest the potential for an increased risk.

It is imperative to perform a medical history and physical examination. A good history can reveal much information. Based on the medical assessment, the practitioner can select the appropriate management, which would include a determination as to what level of anesthesia may be selected and the location at which the treatment would be provided. The diminished reserve associated with aging and the increased sensitivity to anesthetic agents with the potential for the anesthetic depth to deepen rapidly in the geriatric patient do not preclude the geriatric patient from being managed in the office. It simply reinforces the need for very deliberate titration and having patience for the onset of anesthetic effect combined with vigilant monitoring. The greater concern in the geriatric patient is the effect of the patient's comorbidities and medications on anesthetic management, but with an appropriate medical assessment an appropriate anesthetic plan determining anesthetic depth and location can be implemented.

Oral and maxillofacial surgery accreditation standards recognize the unique challenges in anesthetically managing a pediatric patient establishing a minimal number of anesthetic experiences in patients less than 18 years of age. The weakness in this standard is the lack of understanding of what age should define the pediatric patient. The anesthetic management of the pediatric patient differs from that of the geriatric patient, in whom a "lighter" anesthetic depth can provide comfort, analgesia, and improved hemodynamic stability for the geriatric patient but no so for the pediatric patient. Charles J. Cote, MD, asserted that "pediatric conscious sedation is an oxymoron for children younger than 6 years old."[34] An interpretation of this statement to avoid ambiguity if such exists would read: that to anesthetize the younger patient, establishing a child who is cooperative requires either deep sedation or general anesthesia. Once the child has reached 12 years of age, the physiologic and anatomic differences with an adult are less profound, and the differences have a significantly reduced impact on anesthetic care. One could demonstrate that, by the age of 8 or 10 years, the physiologic and anatomic characteristics that were of concern in the pediatric patient have developed such that they are less problematic. Although the OMSNIC data do not demonstrate an increased incidence of morbidity and mortality in the young child, is it intuitive that a standard mandating increased anesthetic training in the pediatric patient should focus on the younger child and not the individual approaching 18 years of age. Additionally, if we accept that a minimum number of cases are required to obtain credentials to sedate the pediatric patient, should there not be a minimum number of cases that are routinely performed on a yearly basis? What is appropriate and/or inadequate to maintain the practitioner's and anesthesia team's competency? I would suggest that 1 case per month would be inadequate, although 2 or more cases per week may not be required. The established anesthetic team model can provide the highest quality of care; however, should there be consideration with selected situations in which a second oral and maxillofacial surgeon or highly trained anesthetic provider should be considered based on the patient age, systemic health, or complexity of surgery. An insistence on incontrovertible proof before making changes to improve patient safety is inaction, which may be counterproductive and detrimental. There is the need for continuance of office-based ambulatory anesthesia care to the pediatric and geriatric patient as delivered by oral and maxillofacial surgery. Oral and maxillofacial surgery has proudly excelled in office-based ambulatory anesthesia and the profession should lead in recommending and establishing the appropriate guidelines.

CONTINUITY OF CARE

There are many components to patient care from the initial consultation to the actual surgery to the postoperative period. Practice dynamics are changing. Whether in the hospital or in an office environment, the patient may be cared for by several practitioners. The patient may see 1 doctor for a consult, a different for the actual procedure, and yet another is on-call and responsible for patient care after the surgery.

The change in practice to limit work hours in the hospital and the partnering of many doctors whether from the same practice or cross-covering from regional practices to provide "off-duty" time for the doctor can negatively impact continuity of care. As the patient traverses the different stages in care, it is critical to ensure appropriate communication between practitioners to minimize the occurrence of errors. Miscommunication during the transference of patient care ("hand-off") has been identified to be contributory to the adverse event in 49% of the cases with a negative outcome.[35]

Contributing factors may comprise the following. Doctors from the same practice may not have the same thoroughness in patient assessment. Furthermore, they may document information differently. This difference may be complicated further when multiple offices are involved using different electronic medical records. To assist with continuity of care, a template that incorporates all critical aspects of care and can be viewed by each doctor can minimize errors. To further minimize errors the system must anticipate and identify discrepancies in care and alert the health care team. Additionally, each doctor must still be responsible for obtaining his or her own information and cannot blindly assume that his or her colleague's information is complete and accurate. Although technological advancements can facilitate information sharing, the success of the system depends the culture of the office. As with many of the points discussed in this article and throughout this issue, a culture of acceptance to new concepts is critical for compliance and actual changes to occur.

Patient care may also be affected by clinical disagreements between doctors. As more doctors are involved in a patient's care, each of these doctors may have a different opinion. There is a greater likelihood for differences in clinical judgment as the patient's medical history increases in complexity. Clinical disagreements between doctors has been reported to be approximately 10% in 1 hospital study and, when such disagreements between doctors exist, there is a greater potential for negative outcomes.[36]

Last, it is important to engage the patient in their care to ensure their own safety. This concept may not be achievable with all patients, because individual patients' health literacy and understanding may vary. However, for many patients and their families there is an understanding of the medical conditions and the frailties that may be associated with the patient's disease. The diabetic patient depicts such a disease. The disease is frequently long-standing and the patient and/or patient family should have some understanding of the disease, basic disease management, and the potential for significant complications with mismanagement. The disease poses preoperative, intraoperative, and postoperative risks that can be minimized by active cooperative and management by both patient and health care provider. The patient or patient's family's role in postoperative care is monitoring blood sugar and contacting the doctor or seeking medical assistance if the patient cannot take adequate oral intake or has unsatisfactory glycemic control. Good postoperative instructions can facilitate that the patient and their family know exactly how they can participate in the patient's care minimizing adverse events. The practitioner can also optimize care by contacting the patient a few hours after discharge from the office whether that be late afternoon or early evening to ensure minimal nausea and vomiting, adequate oral intake, and acceptable glycemic control.

SUMMARY

The intent of this article was not to put blame on an individual. Oral and maxillofacial surgery residency is 4 to 6 years. The majority of surgeons achieve diplomat status in the American Board of Oral and Maxillofacial Surgery. Maintaining diplomat status for those who completed training after 1990 requires recertification every 10 years. There is obviously a clear commitment to excellence and a desire to provide care of the highest quality to the patient by most of our colleagues. No practitioner desires to do harm to his or her patient.

Atul Gawande in his book, *Better: A Surgeon's Notes on Performance*, in the chapter entitled "Bell Curve" explores what differentiates patient outcome of one practitioner from another.[37] In this article, we find that the difference is not necessarily associated with a practitioner's knowledge, but rather with the doctor's attentiveness to detail and critical examination of every aspect of patient care. It is critical to avoid getting trapped in the status quo, such that the eyes and the mind are not open to see and understand what is new and may be important. Average is not bad, if the standard is set high. However, what is unacceptable, is to be satisfied with average and not to strive to do better; "getting better" entails the ability to analyze new concepts and integrate them into one's practice.

REFERENCES

1. Quock RL, Al-Sabbagh M, Mason MK, et al. The dentist as doctor: a rallying call for the future. Oral Surg Oral Med Oral Pathol Oral Radiol 2014; 118(6):637–41.
2. Baum BJ. Inadequate training in the biological sciences and medicine for dental students: an impending crisis for dentistry. J Am Dent Assoc 2007;138: 16–25.
3. Dennis MJ, Bennett JD, DeLuke DM, et al. Improving the medical curriculum in predoctoral dental education: recommendations from the American Association of Oral and Maxillofacial Surgeons Committee on predoctoral education and training. Oral Maxilofacial Surg 2017;75(2):240–4.
4. Wachter RM. The nature and frequency of medical errors and adverse events. In: Wachter RM, editor. Understanding patient safety. New York: McGraw-Hill Companies; 2012. p. 3–19.
5. Qato DM, Wilder J, Schumm LP, et al. Changes in prescription and over-the-counter medication and dietary supplement use among older adults in the United States, 2005 vs 2011. JAMA Intern Med 2016;176:473.
6. Wu CH, Wang CC, Kennedy J. Changes in herb and dietary supplement use in the U.S. adult population: a comparison of the 2002 and 2007 National Health Interview Surveys. Clin Ther 2011;33:1749.
7. Kaufman DW, Kelly JP, Rosenberg L, et al. Recent patterns of medication use in the ambulatory adult population of the United States: the Slone survey. JAMA 2002;287:337.
8. Febbo A, Cheng A, Stein B, et al. Postoperative bleeding following dental extractions in patients anticoagulated with warfarin. J Oral Maxillofac Surg 2016;74(8):1518–23.
9. Elad S, Marshall J, Meyerowitz C, et al. Novel anticoagulants: general overview and practical considerations for dental practitioners. Oral Dis 2016;22:23.
10. Sadeghi-Ghahrody M, Yousefi-Malekshah SH, Karimi-Sari H, et al. Bleeding after tooth extraction in patients taking aspirin and clopidogrel (Plavix®) compared with healthy controls. Br J Oral Maxillofac Surg 2016;54:568.
11. West DR, James KA, Fernald DH, et al. Laboratory medicine handoff gaps experienced by primary care practices: a report from the shared networks of collaborative ambulatory practices and partners (SNOCAP). J Am Board Fam Med 2017;27:796.
12. Graber ML, Franklin N, Gordon R. Diagnostic error in internal medicine. Arch Intern Med 2005;165: 1493.
13. Domino KB, Posner KL, Caplan RA, et al. Airway injury during anesthesia: a closed claims analysis. Anesthesiology 1999;91:1703.

14. Metzner J, Kent CD. Ambulatory surgery: is the liability risk lower? Curr Opin Anaesthesiol 2012;25:654.

15. Wagley C, Hackett C, Haug RH. The effect of preoperative ondansetron on the incidence of postoperative nausea and vomiting in patients undergoing outpatient dentoalveolar surgery and general anesthesia. J Oral Maxillofac Surg 1999;57:1195.

16. Bowater RJ, Stirling SA, Lilford RJ. Is antibiotic prophylaxis in surgery a generally effective intervention? Testing a generic hypothesis over a set of meta-analyses. Ann Surg 2009;249:551.

17. Lodi G, Figini L, Sardella A, et al. Antibiotics to prevent complications following tooth extractions. Cochrane Database Syst Rev 2012;(11):CD003811.

18. Esposito M, Grusovin MG, Worthington HV. Interventions for replacing missing teeth: antibiotics at dental implant placement to prevent complications. Cochrane Database Syst Rev 2013;(7):CD004152.

19. Andreasen JO, Jensen SS, Schwartz O, et al. A systematic review of prophylactic antibiotics in the surgical treatment of maxillofacial fractures. J Oral Maxillofac Surg 2006;64:1664.

20. Alexander JW, Solomkin JS, Edwards MJ. Updated recommendations for control of surgical site infections. Ann Surg 2011;253:1082.

21. Moore PA, Wiffen PJ, Derry S, et al. Non-prescription (OTC) oral analgesics for acute pain: an overview of Cochrane reviews. Cochrane Database Syst Rev 2015;(11):CD010794.

22. Hersh EV, Kane WT, O'Neil MG, et al. Prescribing recommendations for the treatment of acute pain in dentistry. Compend Contin Educ Dent 2011;32:22.

23. Hersh EV, Moore PA, Ross GL. Over-the-counter analgesics and antipyretics: a critical assessment. Clin Ther 2000;22:500.

24. Derry C, Derry S, Moore RA, et al. Single dose ibuprofen for acute postoperative pain in adults. Cochrane Database Syst Rev 2009;(3):CD001548.

25. Jackson DL, Moore PA, Hargreaves KM. Preoperative nonsteroidal anti-inflammatory medication for the prevention of postoperative dental pain. J Am Dent Assoc 1989;119:641.

26. Moore PA, Derry S, Aldington D, et al. Adverse events associated with single dose oral analgesics for acute postoperative pain in adults: an overview of Cochrane reviews. Cochrane Database Syst Rev 2015;(10):CD011407.

27. Gordon SM, Brahim JS, Dubner R, et al. Attenuation of pain in a randomized trial by suppression of peripheral nociceptive activity in the immediate postoperative period. Anesth Analg 2002;95:1351.

28. Moore PA, Dionne RA, Cooper SA, et al. Why do we prescribe Vicodin? J Am Dent Assoc 2016;147:530.

29. Manchikanti L, Helm S II, Fellows B, et al. Opioid epidemic in the United States. Pain Physician 2012;15:ES9–38.

30. Shi A, Rice JB, Kirson NY, et al. Sources of prescription opioids among diagnosed opioid abusers. Curr Med Res Opin 2015;31:779.

31. Voepel-Lewis T, Wagner D, Tait AR. Leftover prescription opioids after minor procedures: an unwitting source for accidental overdose in children. JAMA Pediatr 2015;169:497.

32. McCauley JL, Hyer M, Ramakrishnan VR, et al. Dental opioid prescribing and multiple opioid prescriptions among dental patients. J Am Dent Assoc 2016;147:537.

33. Bennett J, Kramer KJ, Bosack RC. How safe is deep sedation or general anesthesia used while performing dental care? J Am Dent Assoc 2015;146(9):705–8.

34. Cote CJ, Notterman DA, Karl HW, et al. Adverse sedation events in pediatrics: a critical incident analysis of contributing factors. Pediatrics 2000;105:805.

35. Greenberg C, Regenbogen S, Studdert D, et al. Patterns of communication breakdowns resulting in injury to surgical patients. J AM Coll Surg 2007;204:533.

36. Hilsden R, Moffat B, Knowles S, et al. Surgeon agreement at the time of handover, a prospective cohort study. World J Emerg Surg 2016;11:11.

37. Gawande A. Bell curve in a Gawande better. New York: Picador; 2007. p. 201–30.

Proper Management of Medications to Limit Errors

What the Oral Surgeon Should Know to Limit Medication Errors and Adverse Drug Events

Daniel S. Sarasin, DDS[a],*, Jarom E. Mauer, DMD[b]

KEYWORDS

- Adverse drug events • Medication errors • Medication safety • Anesthesia
- Oral and maxillofacial surgery • Perioperative

KEY POINTS

- Perioperative medication errors and adverse drug events occur in OMFS offices.
- The incidence of perioperative medication errors and adverse drug events in oral surgery is unknown.
- Reduction of medication errors and adverse drug events improves anesthesia safety in OMFS.
- Many perioperative medication safety strategies can be used to reduce errors.
- The perioperative medication safety paradigm introduced in this article can improve anesthesia safety in oral surgery offices.

Optimal outcome for patients is the goal every oral and maxillofacial surgeon desires. For decades, the profession has provided anesthesia services in ambulatory settings to alleviate anxiety and discomfort during surgery. The delivery of safe anesthesia and pain control is an essential element to provide quality care. Despite the best intentions anesthesia complications occur. Two of the most common contributing factors are medication errors (MEs) and adverse drug events (ADEs), which can result in morbidity and mortality. Prevention and early identification of these issues are of paramount importance.

DEFINITION OF MEDICATION ERROR AND ADVERSE DRUG EVENT

Not every ME leads to an ADE. Conversely, not all ADEs are caused by MEs. A clear understanding of the definitions of an ME and ADE is important. ME are defined as the failure of a planned action to be completed as intended or the use of a wrong plan to achieve an aim.[1] It is an error in medication prescribing, dispensing, administration, or monitoring the effects of a medication. ADE is an injury caused by medication use.[2] Events that are unpredictable include idiosyncratic or allergic responses. Those that are predictable and potentially avoidable

Disclosure Statement: The authors have nothing to disclose.

[a] Private Practice, Cedar Rapids Oral Surgery and Implant Center, 835 3rd Avenue Southeast, Cedar Rapids, IA 52403, USA; [b] Private Practice, Eastern Iowa Oral and Maxillofacia Surgery, 835 3rd Avenue Southeast, Cedar Rapids, IA 52403, USA

* Corresponding author.

E-mail address: d.sarasin@mchsi.com

include MEs and side effects or toxic reactions that are related to the inherent pharmacologic properties of the drug.

IDENTIFYING AND MANAGING MEDICATION ERRORS AND ADVERSE DRUG EVENTS IN HEALTH CARE

MEs and ADEs are key global public health concerns, which have been written about extensively. These issues are commonly seen across a variety of health care settings. Morbidity and mortality rates and financial costs are staggering. In the past 20 years, there has been dramatic growth in the fields of ME and ADE studies in medicine.[3] One can only extrapolate the medical research findings because dental literature on these subjects is sparse. Dental/oral and maxillofacial surgery (OMFS) patients are unlikely insulated from these problems.

Numerous safety initiatives have been postulated and implemented to reduce the incidence of MEs and ADEs in medicine. Published studies have shown that many of the efforts seem to have improved patient safety in hospital and outpatient settings. Various methods were used to assess the incidence of MEs and ADEs, which included self-reporting, chart review, and direct observation. The accuracy of these assessment tools varies greatly in identifying problems. This issue is evident when one looks at a study by Flynn and colleagues,[4] where 2557 doses of medication were administered on a hospital ward, detection of 456 MEs occurred by direct observation, 34 by chart review, and only one by self-reporting. The validity and reliability of many of these ME and ADE studies have been questioned because of assessment methods used. For one to understand the true impact of safety measures implemented to reduce MEs and ADEs, one must be able to accurately determine their occurrence.

There has clearly been a reduction in MEs and ADEs in many hospitals and medical outpatient clinics globally for several reasons. ME and ADE rates and determination of causes were more closely followed in health care settings. Safety initiatives were developed, implemented, and monitored for effectiveness. Medication administration is now performed following multiple nursing checks. Technologic safety advances are being used, including computerized physician ordering systems with decision support, bar code scanning systems for medication administration, and electronic prescribing systems.[5] In addition, clinical practice agreements were formed between pharmacists and doctors to improve medication safety.[6]

MEDICATION ERRORS AND ADVERSE DRUG EVENTS IN ANESTHESIA

Anesthesia is not immune to these issues. The perioperative setting presents unique patient safety challenges not seen in other areas in the hospital. In 1978, Cooper and colleagues[7] first identified perioperative MEs by retrospective critical-incident analysis. The actual perioperative incidence rates are unknown; the best available data indicate MEs are not rare. Most of these problems have been identified by self-reporting and retrospective evaluation. In an anesthesia closed claims Canadian study by Orser and Byrick,[8] 52% of adverse events were the result of MEs. The operating rooms are one of the only health care settings that have not undergone vigorous ME and ADE assessment. In addition, many of the medication safety methods used in other areas of the hospital, as described in the previous paragraph, are not widely used.

Recently, in a landmark study by Nanji and colleagues[5] investigators performed a randomized prospective observational clinical trial using anesthesia-trained study staff in a tertiary hospital known as a world leader in medication safety. In addition, a retrospective chart review was performed to identify events that were missed by observation. The primary goal of the study was to determine the perioperative incidence of MEs and ADEs. Approximately 1 in 20 medication administrations and every second surgery resulted in an ME and/or an ADE. More than one-third of the errors caused patient harm, whereas the other errors had the potential for harm. There was no significant difference in ME rates for general anesthesia versus sedation-only operations.

TYPES OF MEDICATION ERRORS IN ANESTHESIA

There are many steps involved in the process of perioperative medication administration: (1) the medication is ordered or obtained from the anesthesia cart or from the medication dispensing system; (2) the drug is then dispensed by a pharmacist or withdrawn from the dispensing system; (3) the drug is prepared (eg, withdrawing it from the vial, diluting the medication, and labeling the syringe); (4) the medication is administered; (5) the medication and dosage is documented in the anesthesia record; and (6) the patient is monitored (eg, vital signs, relevant laboratory studies). Frequently, the anesthesia provider is responsible for all these steps. It seems like a simple process, but is more complex when one focuses on the numerous stages. In addition, MEs can occur at any of these steps resulting in ADEs or potential ADEs. There are many types of perioperative MEs (**Box 1**).

Some types of errors are clear, whereas others need to be expounded on. Labeling errors are common, which include no label on the syringe, and incorrect/incomplete information on the label (ie, wrong drug and/or concentration, missing date and time of preparation/expiration on the syringe/vial). A label should be placed on a syringe immediately after filling it.

The incorrect dosage of a drug results in under-dosing or overdosing of a medication. This may be caused by different concentrations of a drug readily available with similar packaging, changing in vendors/brands, inadequate understanding in regards to the pharmacokinetics/pharmacodynamics of a medication as it relates to each patient (ie, correct dose and maximum dose), and calculation errors.

The issue of calculation errors causing incorrect dosage was shown in an observational study by Avidan and colleagues,[9] when they examined the accuracy for anesthesia faculty and residents to calculate pediatric weight-based amount of drug and corresponding amount in milliliters to be drawn from a standard vial to be added to a 50-mL syringe to reach a specific infusion rate. There was no significant difference between the anesthesia personnel groups. Only 15% reached the correct answer. Sixty-one percent of participants had significant calculated errors, where the drug concentrations ranged from 50 times too low up to 56 times too high; an additional 12% of participants calculated the correct total amount of drug but miscalculated the amount of solution to be drawn from the vial. This study did not involve actual patients.

The term improper drug management covers a wide variety of medication issues. These issues include inadvertent or intentional use of a multidose vial on more than one patient, leaving a vial or syringe of a controlled substance left unattended, and improper storage/disposal of a medication. Improper drug management can cause direct harm to patients. In addition, it can cause drug diversion of a controlled substance.

MEDICATION ERROR AND ADVERSE DRUG EVENTS CONTRIBUTING FACTORS

In the past, when an ME or ADE occurred and was identified, a critical analysis would often be undertaken to determine the root cause. Frequently, the finding of the inquiry would be human error and the inquiry would end. More recently, when a human error is identified, further evaluation is performed to determine if the human error is a symptom of deeper, more extensive issues within the organization. Extensive data collection is done to recreate the situation. At that point, given all the information available, factors that contributed to errors are identified. Several studies have looked at factors that contribute to MEs.[10–12] **Box 2** is a compilation of contributing factors reported in the literature.

Drug shortages occur more frequently because of the increased number of drug recalls. Unexpected and unfamiliar drugs and concentrations of drugs may temporarily replace the standard drugs. The term "look alike sound alike drugs" delineates a confusion of medication caused by similar labeling and packaging of different drugs or similar labeling or packaging of the same name but differing concentrations. In the study by Nanji and colleagues,[5] they found patients administered more than 12 medications during anesthesia had more MEs and ADEs.

Box 1
Types of perioperative medication errors

Labeling error

Incorrect dose

Omitted or extra dose of drug

Wrong drug

Wrong timing

Inadvertent bolus

Wrong route

Improper drug management

Box 2
Factors that can contribute to MEs and ADEs

Distraction

Haste/stress/outside pressure

Fatigue/long surgery

Inadequate knowledge

Inadequate communication

Inadequate patient information

Look alike/sound alike drugs

Misread vial or label on syringe

Unexpected/unfamiliar drug

Calculation errors

Severity of patient comorbidity

High number of drugs administered

Reducing the Incidence of Perioperative Medication Errors and Adverse Drug Events

To reduce MEs and ADEs, there must be a heightened awareness of these issues, and a revision of medication safety education for all personnel involved in perioperative anesthesia care. It must be realized that the operating room is a complex environment, where administration of a multitude of potent intravenous medications quickly occurs, often with a limited infrastructure to prevent MEs. This is in direct contrast to other hospital settings, where there are many medication safety measures in place. Multiple safety initiatives have been proposed. They need to be studied and implemented to effectively improve patient safety and avoid the potential for anesthesia personnel to be distracted from other vital tasks.[13]

Safety strategies include technology-based and process-based interventions. Point-of-care bar code–assisted anesthesia document systems, specific drug decision support, electronically controlled "smart" infusion devices containing a drug library, and alerts are examples of technology-based interventions. Changing the timing of medication documentation, connecting infusions to the most proximal intravenous port, and use of prefilled/premixed syringes and infusions prepared by the pharmacy are examples of process-based interventions. If interventions are believed to be cumbersome or ineffective, they will not be universally accepted and methods to bypass these safety devices will persist.

An initiative that seems to address many types of the perioperative MEs was published in 2010 by the Anesthesia Patient Safety Foundation (APSF).[14] The new paradigm that was developed includes four general elements: (1) standardization, (2) technology, (3) pharmacy/prefilled/premixed, and (4) culture. A video on this medication safety paradigm is found on the APSF Web site at www.apsf.org. This four-pronged approach is illustrated in **Box 3**.

For widespread clinical compliance, the safety systems/processes and standardizations must be realistic, practical, and effective. Health care organizations and their facilities are critical to reduce MEs. They also provide moral support to do the correct thing and financial support to help make it happen. Implementation of safety strategies especially technologic-based initiatives is costly. Some safety measures have minimal costs. They include attempts to minimize distractions and interruptions[15]; the use of closed loop communication;

Box 3
STPC paradigm to improve medication safety in the operating room

Standardization

- High-alert drugs (eg, phenylephrine and epinephrine) should be available in standardized concentrations/diluents prepared by pharmacy in ready-to-use (bolus or infusion) form for adult and pediatric patients. Infusions should be delivered by an electronically controlled smart device containing a drug library.
- Ready-to-use syringes and infusions should have standardized fully compliant machine-readable labels.

Technology

- Every anesthesia location should have a mechanism to identify medications before drawing up or administering them (bar code reader) and a mechanism to provide feedback, decision support, and documentation (automated information system).

Pharmacy/Prefilled/Premixed

- Routine provider-prepared should be discontinued whenever possible.
- Clinical pharmacists should be part of the perioperative/operating room team.
- Standardized preprepared medication kits by case type should be used whenever possible.

Culture

- Establish a "just culture" for reporting errors (including near misses) and discussion of lessons learned.
- Establish a culture of education, understanding, and accountability via required curriculum and CME and dissemination of dramatic stories in the *APSF Newsletter* and education videos.
- Establish a culture of cooperation and recognition of the benefits of STPC within and between institutions, professional organizations, and accreditation agencies.

Abbreviation: STPC, standardization, technology, pharmacy/prefilled/premixed, and culture.

and use of medication calculation aids, such as a nomogram for calculating the maximum dose of a drug,[16] pediatric emergency drug calculator that calculates the appropriate dosages of commonly used emergency drugs, maximum dosage of local anesthetics, maximum fluid volumes, and defibrillation settings.[17]

ANESTHESIA MEDICATION ERRORS AND ADVERSE DRUG EVENTS IN ORAL AND MAXILLOFACIAL SURGERY

There is a paucity of literature on anesthesia MEs and ADEs in oral surgery and dentistry except for case reports. The incidence of MEs and resultant or potential ADEs are unknown. One can only extrapolate information, including incidence of these problems, from medical anesthesia studies. The most common method used to identify these issues is self-reporting, which has been shown to miss many of the problems that actually occur. Oral surgery anesthesia studies similar to Nanji and colleagues[5] must be done to determine the true extent of MEs and ADEs in offices. These issues can and do occur in offices; efforts to heighten awareness for the profession is of vital importance. Medication safety education for all oral maxillofacial surgeons and their staff is essential. An editorial by Assael in 2007[18] discusses National Patient Safety Goals as established by the Joint Commission on Accreditation of Health Care Organizations and identifies some medication safety issues that are applicable to oral surgery facilities. Unfortunately, his editorial effort seems to have fallen short of what is necessary: widespread changes in medication safety in offices. When one compares what was done 10 years ago with what is done now in facilities in regards to medication safety little has changed. It must be a priority to reduce MEs and ADEs for patients. Medication safety in oral surgery lags far behind most health care settings including operating rooms.

One must assume that the types of perioperative MEs and actual or potential ADEs that are occurring in OMFS offices are similar to those occurring in the hospital operating rooms (**Box 4**).

REDUCING THE INCIDENCE OF ANESTHESIA MEDICATION ERRORS AND ADVERSE DRUG EVENTS IN ORAL AND MAXILLOFACIAL SURGERY OFFICES

OMFS offices may be more complex environments to deliver anesthesia medication safely than other health care settings. Much can be learned from medical anesthesia colleges in their ongoing efforts to improve medication safety in the hospital

---

Box 4
Types of perioperative MEs in OMFS offices

Labeling errors

Incorrect dose

Omitted or extra dose of drug

Wrong drug

Wrong timing

Improper drug management

---

operating rooms and ambulatory surgical centers. OMFS and dental facilities cannot attempt to duplicate all of the safety initiatives proposed and implemented as previously discussed. This includes the APSF medication safety paradigm, because of technologic differences, lack of pharmacy support, and exorbitant cost. The chasm that exists between medicine and OMFS/dentistry health care settings requires one to carefully assess the perioperative medication safety protocols medical anesthesiologists are using, to determine if they are feasible. There are many medication safety initiatives that can be implemented to help address the issue of MEs and ADEs. There are financial costs to some of these initiatives. Improving medication patient safety is not cheap, but patients are worth the expense. Some strategies need to be incorporated into offices, whereas others are in place, but need to be reinforced.

OMFS needs its own anesthesia medication safety paradigm. We introduce a paradigm, which we have developed. This perioperative medication safety paradigm focuses on five general elements that are integral to reducing MEs and ADEs in OMFS and dentistry: (1) improve medication safety education, (2) know the patient, (3) know the medication, (4) proper management of anesthetic agents, and (5) proper management of emergency medication (**Box 5**).

Improve Medication Safety Education

Drug safety must be a top priority. OMFS and dentistry organizations must step up and help

---

Box 5
Perioperative medication safety paradigm for OMFS

Improve medication safety education

Know the patient

Know the drugs

Proper management of anesthetic agents

Proper management of emergency medication

lead. Drug safety education for all members of the operator-anesthetist team (OAT) is essential. Reducing MEs and ADEs must be everyone's goal. The awareness of all members of the OAT must be heightened if the goal is to be reached. Critical assessment of should be done frequently.

Know the Patient

Know the patient to optimize anesthesia care. A thorough preoperative work-up is of paramount importance. A comprehensive history and physical examination, and appropriate referrals is necessary. A list of all medications including recreational drugs and supplements the patient is using and medication allergies must be reviewed. Potential drug interactions with the patient's medications/supplements and proposed anesthetic agents should be reviewed. An anesthesia treatment plan for each patient can then be developed. The alteration of a medication regimen, including adding, switching, holding, or adjusting drug dosages, may be an integral part of the plan. When a drug regimen is modified preoperatively, information must also be provided as to when and how the patient should resume their regular drug regimen after anesthesia. Telling the patient/patient care provider the recommended alteration of the medication regimen is not enough; clearly written instructions/orders must be given before and after anesthesia care.

Developing a clinical practice agreement between a pharmacist and oral surgeon may reduce perioperative MEs and ADEs.

Compliance with recommendations must be checked on the day of treatment (eg, taking their regular medications and/or a prophylactic antibiotic, holding or adjusting an antihyperglycemic or anticoagulant agent). On the day of the treatment, a preoperative assessment must be performed, including updating of the medical history, a reconciliation of the patient's current medication regimen, and a brief physical assessment to determine changes since the initial appointment. Additionally, the anesthesia treatment plan must be reviewed and possibly revised if indicated by recent medical problems and current medical findings.

Know the Drugs

Know the drugs to improve anesthesia outcome. Thorough understanding of the anesthetic agents used in an office is common sense. The knowledge of a drug's action, potential side effects, drug interactions, maximum dose, and appropriate dosage cannot be overstated. Periodic review by the OAT of all medications administered in the office including emergency drugs is important. Before adding a new medication into our office, it is extensively studied and all of the personnel involved with anesthesia patient care are educated in the safe usage of the drug.

Medication pharmacokinetics and pharmacodynamics variations between age groups must be clear to safely administer anesthesia to all patients. The pharmacokinetics of newborns, infants, and children are significantly different than adults; they are not small adults in regards to drug usage. The same is said with the elderly. The differences can predispose each of these patients groups to ADEs and underdosing or overdosing of drugs if the dosages and/or timing of administration are not adjusted. In regards to drug pharmacodynamics, during development (ie, neonates to adolescents) and systemic decline (ie, elderly) neurotransmitters, hormones, and receptors play different roles than adults leading to differing therapeutic response to medications. These differences can influence drug effectiveness and toxicity.

Proper Management of Anesthetic Agents

Proper management of anesthetic agents increases medication safety. Medication management begins with ordering the drugs from vendors and ends with the discarding of unused medication with a multitude of steps in between. Obtaining anesthetics agents and emergency drugs for OMFS facilities usually involves working with a few vendors/pharmacies. Attention to detail is necessary when ordering medications to ensure the proper medications and concentrations are selected. This is especially true when drug recalls occur, because of drug shortages. Frequently other vendors or pharmacies are used and/or other drug concentrations are inadvertently ordered. A conscious effort to limit the number of drugs with more than one concentration in OMFS offices is important.

Careful inspection of the drugs received by the office is required. The concentration of these drugs should be compared with existing drugs in the office to ensure the correct drug concentration. Differing drug concentrations of the same drug can lead to inadvertent underdosing or overdosing. Unintended overheating or freezing of the medication before or during transport can occur. The drug vials should be inspected for damage and contamination. Additionally, storage of medications in a temperature-controlled environment as specified by drug manufacturers is warranted and controlled medications must be stored in a secure location.

The proper preparation of medication is extremely important to reduce MEs and ADEs. This task includes withdrawing it from a vial and labeling the syringes. This should be done in a clean, quiet environment to minimize distractions. The use of a multidose vial of a medication is intended for a single patient; the vial should not be used for more than one patient. Strict sterile technique is essential. Two members of the OAT trained in medication safety should work together during drug preparation. This practice can reduce drug diversion. The medication concentration should be checked on the drug vial to ensure the correct concentration of drug is drawn up. Labels are made and placed on the syringes immediately after the syringes are filled. Information on the drug labels should include the drug name, drug concentration, date/time of drug preparation, and date/time of drug expiration. The use of colored labels for each commonly used medication may reduce the risk of accidental wrong drug administration. Customized medication drug trays can be used to create a well-organized anesthetic workspace. Look alike/sound alike drugs must be intentionally separated. The use of a special label can also be applied to help identify these drugs.

Some offices combine propofol and remifentanil in syringes and administer this mixture with an infusion pump. The separation of these drugs over time will occur. It is essential that the preparation of this drug combination be performed immediately before administration. Delayed use after medication preparation can increase the concentration of one drug, while reducing the concentration of the other drug. In addition, close attention is necessary when combining these medications to ensure the appropriate, intended drug concentrations are formulated.

The administration of a medication and documentation, and monitoring the effects of the drug should occur simultaneously. A concerted effort by all members of the OAT is essential. Everyone needs to be focusing on the same thing: the patient. Attention to details and completion of assigned tasks are essential. An example is monitoring continuous infusion of intravenous fluid. Loss of intravenous access or stopping intravenous infusion of fluid can result in omission or delay of drug administration, unless this issue is immediately identified. The use of closed loop communication reduces communication problems and keeps everyone focused on the patient. It can improve efforts for documentation of medications used and monitoring of the drug's effects on the patient. Institute a critical language protocol for the OAT in which an agreed on term or phrase stops activity. When a member of the team perceives an imminent risk to the patient, a critical phrase is a useful and powerful mechanism to gain attention of all team members and momentarily stops all activity so a group evaluation may be made of the perceived risk. It can also be used in situations where the patient is awake and family members are present. The term should be neutral and avoids causing unnecessary alarm.[19] Reduction of outside distractions and interruption during anesthesia, especially when medication is administered, is essential.

Unused medications need to be immediately and properly discarded after the procedure has ended and the patient is recovering before discharge. This prevents accidental use of a medication on another patient. In addition, it reduces the risk for drug diversion.

Proper Management of Emergency Medication

Proper management of emergency medication reduces morbidity and mortality. A thorough understanding of emergency drugs and periodic review by the OAT team is essential. It should occur more frequently than when the drug is replaced on the expiration date. Relying on the team's cognitive ability to recall vital drug information during an emergency is problematic. Having a small card beside or under the medication vial with information that includes its action, appropriate dose, maximum dose, and indications and contraindications for use is necessary. If a drug requires dilution before administration, a special label should be placed on the drug vial and appropriate protocol for dilution of the drug should be included on the card. The preparation of emergency medications should be practiced regularly by the OAT, especially drugs that require dilution. All members of the OAT should be familiar with the emergency cart and where each drug is located. The drug cart must be organized, with sound alike/look alike medications separated. It is common for two different concentrations of epinephrine to be included in emergency kits. Special labeling and a clear understanding of the indications for each of the epinephrine concentrations are warranted. Drug compartments must be clearly marked. Emergency medications should have their expiration date logged; drugs should be replaced at the time of their expiration date or just prior.

Efforts should be made to simplify drug decisions during an emergency. Anesthesia emergency algorithms can assist the OAT with selecting the appropriate medication and dosage. In addition, it can aid the team in accidently omitting a crucial medication. The use of a pediatric emergency calculator uses the child's weight to calculate various emergency medication dosages. This is routinely printed out before anesthesia in case an emergency arises. Another method commonly used in emergencies is the Broselow tape/strip. This method is less accurate than the pediatric drug calculator because it uses the child's height in determining the appropriate medication dosages instead of body weight.

Proper management of anesthesia emergencies frequently requires emergent administration of drugs. Delays in medication delivery can adversely affect patient outcome. The use of emergency mediation kits that are prepared by hospital pharmacies and contain prefilled/premixed syringes and infusion bags has been shown to reduce medication delivery time and medication preparation, and improve drug standardization. One of the drawbacks to using pharmacy-prepared emergency kits in OMFS facilities is the drugs are often unused and discarded after expiration, which leads to increased costs. Having more commonly used prefilled/premixed medication syringes available instead of an entire emergency medication kit is more practical for OMFS facilities.

IMPLEMENTING A MEDICATION SAFETY PLAN IN AN ORAL AND MAXILLOFACIAL SURGERY FACILITY

The idea of making major changes to reduce MEs and ADEs seems to be a daunting costly task. OMFS offices that have had a recent significant ADE or identified a near miss are likely to be more amenable to change. For many other oral surgeons, they are less inclined to alter their daily anesthesia office routine. It is a matter of human nature. Why change something that is not broken? Or is it broken? In regards to perioperative medication safety (ie, ME and ADE rates), it all comes down to how one looks at the problem, prospectively or retrospectively. Compare the findings from Nanji and colleagues study[5] (1 in 20 perioperative medication administrations had an ME and/or ADE) with Oster and colleagues[20] survey study (85% of anesthesiologist reported at least one drug error or near miss during their careers). The answer is obvious to how our profession/oral surgeons should look at medication safety. Gradual institution of safety initiatives in each area of the perioperative medication safety paradigm illustrated in **Box 5** is likely to improve implementation and compliance by the OAT. Multiple small changes over time are more likely to reduce stress for office staff and are met with less resistance than large sweeping changes. If one wishes for changes to occur, one must be sensitive that change can be difficult. Regular assessment of the newly added medication strategies should be examined before adding additional drug safety initiatives. The OAT compliance to medication safety strategies is often lower that other safety initiatives introduced because the benefits of these programs (ie, reduction in perioperative MEs and ADEs rates) are not obvious. Feedback from the OAT on how things are working and perceived problems that may be associated with the incorporation of these strategies is important. This helps to instill a sense of empowerment for the team. One must be flexible and open to modifying drug safety protocols.

SUMMARY

Providing safe and effective ambulatory anesthesia is a key component to deliver optimal OMFS care for patients. OMFS must focus on medication safety. This article reviews the issue of perioperative MEs and ADEs and introduces a perioperative medication safety paradigm and practical initiatives that can be implemented in OMFS facilities that may help to make the goal of optimal care a reality. Medication safety education and research is necessary and essential.

REFERENCES

1. Kohn LT, Corrigan JM, Donaldson MS. To err is human: building a safer health system. Washington, DC: National Academy Press; 2000.
2. Aspden P, Wolcott J, Bootman JL, et al, editors. Committee on identifying and preventing medication errors. Preventing medication errors: quality chasm series. Washington, DC: National Academy Press; 2007.
3. Huang HC, Wang CH, Chen PC, et al. Bibliometric analysis of medication errors and adverse drug events. J Patient Saf 2015. [Epub ahead of print].
4. Flynn EA, Barker KN, Pepper GA, et al. Comparison of methods for detecting medication errors in 36 hospitals and skilled-nursing facilities. Am J Health Syst Pharm 2002;59:436–46.
5. Nanji KC, Patel A, Shaikh S, et al. Evaluation of perioperative medication errors and adverse drug events. Anesthesiology 2016;124:25–34.
6. Pedersen CA, Schneider PJ, Scheckelhoff DJ. ASHP National survey of pharmacy practice in hospital settings: prescribing and transcribing-2010. Am J Health Syst Pharm 2011;68(8):669–88.
7. Cooper JB, Newbrower RS, Long CD, et al. Preventable anesthesia mishaps: a study of human factors. Anesthesiology 1978;49:399–406.
8. Orser BA, Byrick R. Anesthesia-related medication error: time to take action. Can J Anaesth 2004;51:756–60.
9. Avidan A, Levin PD, Weissman C, et al. Anesthesiologists' ability in calculating weight-based concentrations for pediatric drug infusion: an observational study. J Clin Anes 2014;26:276–80.

10. Webster CS, Merry AF, Larsson L, et al. The frequency and nature of drug administration error during anesthesia. Aneasth Intensive Care 2001;29:494–500.

11. Kahn FA, Hoda MQ. A prospective survey of intraoperative critical incidences in a teaching hospital in a developing country. Anaesthesia 2001;56:177–82.

12. Cooper L, DiGiovanni N, Schultz L, et al. Influences observed on incidence and reporting of medication errors in anesthesia. Can J Anesth 2012;59:562–70.

13. Orser BA, U D, Cohen MR. Perioperative medication errors: building safer system. Anesthesiology 2016; 124(1):1–3.

14. Eichhorn JH. APSF hosts medication safety conference consensus group defines challenges and opportunities for improved practice. APSF Newsl 2010;25(1):1–8.

15. Pape TM, Dingman SK. Interruptions and distractions during anesthesia induction: a pilot study. Plast Surg Nurs 2011;31(2):49–56.

16. Williams DJ, Walker JD. A nomogram for calculating the maximum dose of local anaesthetic. Anaesthesiology 2014;69:847–53.

17. Rollert M. Practical pearl: pediatric emergency drug calculator. Pulse 2016;48(1):17.

18. Assael LA. The need for national patient safety goals for ambulatory oral and maxillofacial surgery. J Oral Maxillofac Surg 2007;65(10):1–2.

19. Frankel A. Patient safety: anesthesia in remote locations. Anesthes Clin 2009;27(1):136.

20. Oster BA, Chen RJ, Tee DA. Medication errors in anesthetic practice: a survey of 687 practitioners. Can J Anaeth 2001;48:139–46.

Preventing Wrong-Site Surgery in Oral and Maxillofacial Surgery

Leon A. Assael, DMD

KEYWORDS

- Patient safety • Surgical checklists • Ambulatory oral surgery • Anesthesia care • Surgical training

KEY POINTS

- The complexity of the clinical tasks required to perform ambulatory oral and maxillofacial surgery has accelerated to the point that errors are inevitable; systems are needed to eliminate wrong-site surgery.
- Among the most valuable and proved methods to mitigate the risks of medical errors has been the development of surgical checklists.
- Although checklists have come slowly to oral and maxillofacial surgery and to other disciplines in dentistry, they may provide exceptional value in the complicated and less regulated environment of ambulatory oral surgical procedures.
- Today, wrong tooth extraction remains a frequent reason for professional liability claim against oral and maxillofacial surgeons.

Wrong surgical site surgery has gained great attention in hospitals and in ambulatory care as part of national patient safety standards efforts. All oral and maxillofacial surgeons working in the operating room have become well aware of these efforts but they have not been consistently incorporated into the ambulatory care setting as yet. This may be due to the incorrectly presumed lesser complexity of the ambulatory setting or the lack of institutional oversight in such settings. In addition, the operating room team is often less developed and less focused on the interprofessional environment in ambulatory care than it is in the hospital operating room setting. Nonetheless, the ambulatory oral and maxillofacial surgery setting faces exactly the same issues as the inpatient setting with regard to patient safety. Thus, it is time for the utility of these measures to be assessed by oral and maxillofacial surgeons and time to adapt their use appropriately to the setting or ambulatory oral and maxillofacial surgery.

These efforts to prevent wrong-site surgery and related complications began when it became common knowledge that deaths, complications, and disfigurement from medical errors were frequent and preventable clinical problems. Because a medical error, wrong-site surgery, is always preventable, mechanisms have been developed and evaluated to mitigate these risks. Among the most valuable and proved methods has been the development of surgical checklists.

Necessary processes must be in place and implemented continuously to prevent wrong-site surgery. Intent to reduce errors alone is not sufficient in reducing risk. To initiate these processes, organizations responsible for health care quality took action. In 2016 the Joint Commission

Division of Oral and Maxillofacial Surgery, Department of Developmental and Surgical Sciences, School of Dentistry, University of Minnesota, 515 Delaware Street, Minneapolis, MN 55455, USA
E-mail address: assael@umn.edu

Oral Maxillofacial Surg Clin N Am 29 (2017) 151–157
http://dx.doi.org/10.1016/j.coms.2016.12.003
1042-3699/17/© 2017 Elsevier Inc. All rights reserved.

released its updated patient safety goals for ambulatory care.[1] It included 2 goals pertinent to wrong-site surgery in oral and maxillofacial surgery. These are to identify patients correctly and to prevent mistakes in surgery:

"NPSG.01.01.01 Use at least two ways to identify patients. For example, use the patient's name and date of birth ..."

"UP.01.01. 01 Make sure that the correct surgery is done on the correct patient and at the correct place on the patient's body"

"UP 01.02.01 Mark the correct place on the patient's body where the surgery is to be done"

"UP 01.03.01 Pause before the surgery to make sure that a mistake is not being made"

These updated elements of Joint Commission goals form the skeleton of surgical checklists. A surgical checklist is simply the means to assess that the Joint Commission goals are being met continuously in the care of every patient and for every medical/surgical intervention.

CAUSES OF WRONG-SITE SURGERY

To understand the value of checklists, it is helpful to reprise the causes of wrong-site surgery. The generic causes of wrong-site surgery have been ascertained and well summarized. Each of these causes is pertinent to the oral and maxillofacial surgery practice.[2] They include

1. The lack of a formal operationalized system to verify the correct patient and site
2. The lack of a checklist
3. The inconsistent use of the checklist
4. The lack of a cohesive surgical team with each team member empowered to assure patient safety
5. High volume of surgical cases or other time pressures
6. The complexity of the surgical site, multiple procedures, and coexisting pathology
7. The use of highly specialized equipment
8. Surgical site visualization
9. Competency and credentialing of the whole surgical team
10. Ability to access proper information on the patient and the planned procedure
11. Development of a coherent treatment plan
12. Patient charting or chart review errors
13. Patient confidentiality and security
14. Adequate staffing
15. Training of the surgical team
16. Culture of the surgical team
17. Multiple surgeons/physicians/dentists with pass-off miscommunication
18. Nonmarked surgical site or surgical site marking error
19. Miscommunication with the patient or responsible party
20. Not systematically reviewing the checklist during a preprocedure pause

Specific comment regarding the pertinence of this list to the oral and maxillofacial surgery team is notable. The ambulatory setting in oral and maxillofacial surgery has not traditionally included a checklist. A cohesive and well-trained clinical team is variable in that in some states, licensure and credentialing of dental assistants are not required. Although the specialized education of the surgical team toward oral surgery has been well promulgated by the American Association of Oral and Maxillofacial Surgeons through the Dental Anesthesia Assistant National Certification Examination (DAANCE) program, its use is variably regulated.[3] In addition, the DAANCE program focuses on basic sciences, evaluation of patients with systemic diseases, anesthetic drugs, monitoring, and emergencies. It does not focus on the national patient safety standards that are part of continuing education in the interprofessional hospital setting. Although this could be accomplished as part of allied health professions education, the only educational requirement for participation in DAANCE is Basic Life Support certification. The educational requirements to perform duties as part of the surgical team in ambulatory oral and maxillofacial surgery differ substantially from those in the hospital operating room. These differences in education create additional challenges toward achieving the national patient safety goals of the Joint Commission on Accreditation of Health Care Organizations (JCACO).

In addition, the oral surgery ambulatory clinical team can be variably educated and with a high turnover rate. The culture of the oral and maxillofacial surgery team can be different from that of the operating room. The empowerment of all team members to participate fully in the care of patients is variable. The consulting surgeon and the operating surgeon might be 2 different members of a group practice. Surgical sites are not typically marked. The treatment rendered is often not part of a cohesive/comprehensive treatment plan. Visualization of the surgical site in the oral cavity may be difficult. Miscommunication with the patient who may be sedated or given an anxiolytic is a source of error. There is typically no pause before initiating the procedure. From this overview, it is clear that the ambulatory oral and maxillofacial surgery environment faces special challenges in addressing these 20 causes of wrong-site surgery and that change in the administration of ambulatory oral and maxillofacial surgery care is needed to accomplish these goals.

UTILITY FOR ORAL AND MAXILLOFACIAL SURGERY

Although checklists have come slowly to oral and maxillofacial surgery and to other disciplines in dentistry, they may provide exceptional value in the complicated and less regulated environment of ambulatory oral surgical procedures. Wrong-site surgery has been a perennial endemic problem in oral and maxillofacial surgery practice, particularly in exodontia.[4] According to insurers, in 2007, 14% of all oral surgery claims were for wrong-site surgery whereas only 2% of all orthopedic claims were for wrong-site surgery.[5]

Today, wrong tooth extraction remains a frequent reason for professional liability claim against oral and maxillofacial surgeons. For a visible anatomic structure with visible pathology in most cases, it is worth examining why this is so. The 52 deciduous and permanent teeth (and supernumerary teeth) involved in a prescription for exodontia, the nature of referrals for exodontia, various numberings systems not accepted under universal nomenclature, wrong-side errors due to mounting of nondigital radiographs, the ubiquitous nature of dental diseases, the inability of patients to have a detailed understanding of their own dental anatomy and pathology, the diffuse and poorly localized nature of odontalgia, the similar anatomic features of teeth that have drifted in the arch, and economic barriers to clinical decision making as well as the usual cultural and communication barriers in all clinical encounters are some of the reasons that exodontia might be a surgical procedure particularly prone to wrong-site surgery error. Some detailed explanation of these causes is considered.

The 52 teeth have variable and continuous anatomic characteristics in terms of coronal and root anatomy. Teeth migrate or can be in ectopic position and are often declared different teeth by 2 clinicians seeing the same patient. This is particularly true for first, second, and third molars where errors seem more frequent, especially after the prior loss of a molar.

The nature of referrals for exodontia is such that a comprehensive oral diagnosis may not have been completed by the referring provider. Incomplete clinical assessment and radiographic evaluation often results in disparities in diagnostic assessment. Numbering systems and marking of referral charts are often sources of error.

Numbering systems of teeth, the nomenclature of their identity, vary globally and by practice custom. Not every school, payer, dental specialty, nation, or individual uses the same numbering system. For all teeth, the following numbering systems are in use. The universal numbering system (also known as the universal notation system and as the American system), numbers teeth 1 to 32, beginning in the maxillary right third molar and continuing in sequence through the maxilla right to left, and, beginning with tooth 17 (mandibular left third molar), completing the arch in the right mandibular third molar with tooth number 32. In addition, the 20 deciduous teeth are labeled right to left in the maxilla and left to right in the mandible with tooth numbers A–T. Not surprisingly, this arcane system with no intuitive basis is prone to error. It is only used in the United States due to historical reasons. This system is particularly prone to producing right-left errors as well as errors in planning deciduous tooth extraction because no guidance other than memorization is given to selecting the dental arch or side of extraction.

The International Organization for Standardization (ISO) system (also known as the World Dental Federation/Fédération Dentaire International [FDI] system and as the World Health Organization [WHO] system) is a 2-digit system developed to address these issues. In the ISO system, the first digit identifies the quadrant: upper right is quadrant 1, upper left quadrant 2, lower left 3, and lower right 4. The quadrants, however, are renamed 5 to 8 for deciduous teeth. The second digit identifies the tooth number in the quadrant from anterior to posterior, 1 to 8 for permanent and 1 to 5 for deciduous teeth. A third system, which preceded the others, is the Zsigmondy/Palmer notation system, in which a bracket is used to identify the quadrant, such as "L" for upper left quadrant and "⌉" for the mandibular right quadrant, and 1 to 8 used for permanent and A–E for deciduous teeth. Thus a mandibular right third molar is "8⌉."[6]

To compound nomenclature confusion, teeth with different numbering systems can have identical numbers but indicate different teeth. For example, in the American system, tooth number 16 is the maxillary left third molar, but in the ISO system it is the maxillary right first molar. Without attesting to the system used, errors in pass-off of treatment plans may result. This is a problem observed even during examinations, because American dental students attempt to take international examinations, such as for licensure in Canada. Perhaps in an attempt to obviate this problem, it is recommended that 16 in the ISO system be stated as "one-six" rather than "sixteen."

The mounting of nondigital radiographs relies on a bump on the film to indicate the front or an "L" for left on panoramic radiograph. When copied, the site markings or bump are often not transferred and when mounted the bump may not be palpable. When placed on a view box, the "L" is often hidden. In addition, not all clinicians mount radiographs in the customary fashion, as if they were looking at the patient, for example, left side mounted on right side of the mounting frame.

The ubiquitous nature of dental diseases, caries and periodontal diseases are systems-based ailments that normally affect multiple structures simultaneously. The visible ailment may not reflect the current state of advancing pathology. There are limits of odontalgia as a predictive diagnostic symptom. Referred pain and poorly localized pain can vary over time and might create evolving symptoms temporally variable during diagnosis. In addition, nonodontologic pathology, such as sinusitis, neuralgia, or myofascial pain, can lead to misdiagnosis of odontologic cause of symptoms.

Patients have a limited understanding of their own dental structures. Relying on patients to explain their diagnosis and the planned procedure can often produce error in oral surgery and in other surgical practice as well. Patients may be insistent over their desired procedure at variance to the treatment plan or surgeon's own assessment.

Tooth drifting and ectopic position, such as in removal for orthodontic purposes, may result in error because the tooth should be prescribed for extraction based on its anatomy, not on its location in the arch. Incorrect removal of first premolars for orthodontic purpose is a risk when removal of second premolars is recommended because the routine expectation for removal plan by the surgeon is at variance with the prescribed plan.

Economic barriers in clinical decisions: the costs of care due to a logical treatment plan based on extant pathology is often not offered for the exodontia patient. Simply put, hopelessly diseased teeth are often not on the clinical request form for extraction due to the costs associated with their removal and replacement. As an example, a visibly nondiseased tooth with pulpitis might be requested for extraction whereas an adjacent hopelessly diseased tooth might not be selected for extraction due to nonmedical economically based decision. This too, can result in extraction of the "wrong tooth" at least vis-à-vis what was prescribed for extraction.

Culture and communication barriers typically associated with the clinical care setting are not as well managed in the ambulatory oral and maxillofacial surgery setting. Most health care organizations have translators immediately available often as required by law. Patient advocates address cultural and social issues in hospitals. Surgical consent may be done with a higher level of rigor, especially by nursing staff in the presurgical area. These systems are not in place in the same fashion in ambulatory oral and maxillofacial surgery.

All these issues point out the need for a patient safety protocol customized for the special environment of ambulatory oral and maxillofacial surgery.

PREVENTION OF WRONG TOOTH EXTRACTION
Education

Protocols for prevention of wrong tooth extraction have been initiated in dental practice and the outcomes of those interventions have been measured. Chang and colleagues[7] reported on the effectiveness of education in reducing this incidence. In the 3 years before the intervention in a single clinic, 8 preventable wrong-site extractions occurred. In each case a root cause analysis was performed, including a committee that assessed the reasons for the occurrence and proposed a program that was initiated for the study period. They identified the following guidelines to prevent wrong tooth extraction: the use of diagnosis (eg, nonrestorable caries) in the extraction order, informing the patient of the location of the tooth being removed and the condition for which it was being removed, and verifying the order for extraction with the patient. This was a simple education program without a checklist. After a training period, there were no wrong tooth extractions in the ensuing 3 years. Although this investigation did not use contemporary standards for prevention of wrong-site surgery, it demonstrates that simply paying attention to detail in rudimentary ways can promote successful outcomes in practice.

Developing the Surgical Team

The culture of the surgical team has been strongly developed in operating rooms and in industry. Lessons from these changes can be incorporated into ambulatory oral surgery practice. In industrial activities, the Japanese concept of kaizen (good change) has been a mainstay.[8] It was known that activities, such as commercial airlines and automotive manufacturing among others, had lower catastrophe rates when all team members were empowered to make changes for continuous improvement. The principles of kaizen are that good change brings good results through understanding circumstances, using data, taking action to correct root causes of problems, working as a team, and empowering every member of the team. These principles have created higher levels of participation and personal investment in outcomes among effective teams. Although clinical team members say they have diminished the role of the leader of the team, in fact they have created a more effective culture of safety.

Checklists

A global initiative to reduce wrong-site surgery and other perioperative complications, such as retained instruments, medical or transfusion error, and avoidable intraoperative complications, has been launched.[9] The WHO launched a program, now available in numerous languages and supported by a teaching manual, to promulgate the WHO Surgical Safety Checklist. Although the first edition remains in 2016, it has been a 10-year effort, beginning with the Safe Surgery Saves Lives project in 2006.[10,11]

The WHO team performed an evidence-based evaluation of the preventable complications related to surgery and determined to focus on the following areas for corrective action planning:

1. Correct site surgery
2. Safe anesthesia care
3. Airway
4. Bleeding
5. Allergies
6. Postoperative infection
7. Foreign body retention
8. Handling of surgical specimens
9. Communication
10. Outcomes assessment

Checklists have been long used in aerospace, naval activities, scientific research, and industrial production, among other areas. Everyone who has ever watched the launch of a spacecraft has witnessed the enormous concurrent effort associated with checklists that must be time dependent and coordinated. The decision to bring checklists into health care was done without direct knowledge as to how they might have an impact on outcomes, but experience from other industries indicated that checklists are a powerful bulwark against the error of omission in complex processes.

The surgical checklist is integrated into the evaluation, assessment, and interventions needed to have an impact on these areas. It is divided into 3 parts: sign in before the induction of anesthesia, time out before the incision, and sign out before the patient leaves the operating room.

Each of these can be review and considered in the context of ambulatory oral and maxillofacial surgery. A reprise of each item in the WHO checklist is listed and with comments on its suitability to the ambulatory oral and maxillofacial surgery setting.[12]

Sign In

1. The patient has confirmed identity, site, procedure, and consent. This can be performed with the patient at the time of final review of the consent form, at which time the patient can confirm identity, location, and procedure for the planned oral procedure
2. Site is marked or deemed not applicable. For typical oral surgical procedures in the visible oral cavity, including extractions, marking the surgical site is practical and can be performed with typical nontoxic surgical marking pens. At the time of marking, the site can also be confirmed with the patient. This is well done with the patient holding a full-face mirror. For quadrant-based dentoalveolar procedures, the site can be marked on the mucosa or overlying skin. For vestibular or other mucosal incisions, the site can be directly marked and demonstrated to the patient. The surgical site is always applicable in the oral surgery setting.
3. Anesthesia safety check is completed. Gas systems, bag-valve mask, endotracheal tubes, laryngoscope, medications, crash cart, hoses, pressure, oxygen sensor, backup gases, monitors, suction, and personnel should all be checked in the oral surgery setting before initiating surgery, including for patients undergoing local anesthesia, nitrous oxide analgesia, conscious sedation, or general anesthesia. In the oral surgery setting, all local anesthesia care is monitored anesthetic care, at least to the extent of providing emergency support
4. Pulse oximetry on patient and is functioning. Preoperative vital signs are a standard of care for all oral surgical procedures but pulse oximetry is not in complete usage for local anesthesia cases. It is required for sedation cases. Oximetry during surgery has become routine for local anesthesia cases in other settings and should be considered in oral surgery based on the stresses of surgery and the considerations for altered airway or cardiovascular status that might occur with surgery in the upper airway.
5. Does the patient have a known allergy? This is both on the checklist and typically recorded on the chart or wall in hospital setting. An

appropriate area of the operatory, anesthesia machine, chalkboard, or wall can be consistently used in the oral surgery setting to inform the entire care team of allergies.

6. Assessment of difficult airway or aspiration risk is performed. When airway risk is noted, the oral surgeon can reposition the patient; make available appropriate airway and laryngoscope; assess the need for surgical field isolation, for example, drape; plan supplemental or specialized suction and irrigation; and apply personnel assistance to mitigate the risk of airway obstruction or aspiration. Sources and type of suction are selected at this time. Assessing the need for and making available a surgical airway must be considered in cases of operative related airway obstruction anticipated.

7. Risk of blood loss is greater than 500 mL or 7 mL/kg in children. The WHO recommends intravenous (IV) access and fluids for such cases. As much as 250 mL blood loss per arch can be anticipated for full mouth extraction with alveoplasty. Patients with bleeding disorders or medication-induced coagulopathies can be anticipated to have greater blood loss, even with good initial hemostasis intraoperatively. The need for IV fluids due to nothing-by-mouth status also needs to be addressed at the time of the checklist. The use of IV fluids in such cases in the ambulatory oral and maxillofacial surgery setting is recommended.

Time Out

The time out is a critical event performed just prior to initiating the surgical procedure in which all aspects of the checklist are confirmed. It includes the following:

1. Confirm that all team members have introduced themselves by name and role.
2. Surgeon anesthesia professional and nurse verbally confirm the patient, the site, and the procedures.
3. Anticipated critical events are noted:
   a. Surgeon reviews the critical or unexpected steps, operative duration, anticipated blood loss.
   b. Anesthesia team reviews any patient specific concerns.
   c. Nursing team reviews sterility confirmed and whether there are any equipment issues or other concerns.
4. Has antibiotic prophylaxis been given with the past 60 minutes?
5. Is essential imaging displayed? A key element in ambulatory oral and maxillofacial surgery is not only whether radiographs are displayed

but also whether they are displayed properly and whether the images displayed are those of the patient and can be confirmed as such.

Sign Out

At the conclusion of the procedure, the following sign-out events occurs:

1. Nurse verbally confirms with the team:
   a. That the name of the procedure is recorded
   b. That instrument sponge and needle counts are correct.
   c. Assure that the specimen is properly labeled
   d. Whether any equipment problems need to be addressed
2. Surgeon anesthesia professional and nurse review the key concerns for recovery and management of this patient.

The importance of the sign out is that it confirms to the surgical team that all aspects of the planned procedure are complete. This is an important step of particular value in the oral surgery setting where incomplete procedures due to the multiple facets of planned procedures are a notable problem. Also essential for the oral surgery team is an understanding of the location and number of surgical hemostatic tamponade packs. All alloplastic materials used, and biologics, lot numbers, and location of inserted devices need to be noted as recorded in the sign out. The location and recording of biopsy specimens are also noted.

The value of patient safety procedures to prevent wrong-site surgery is empirically clear after root cause analysis of failures as well as cohort studies. Most of these cohort studies have occurred in general surgical settings, and there seem to be no randomized clinical trials due to the need to protect human subjects from a randomized intervention/nonintervention study. The outcomes of checklists are clear. The use of a checklist reduces complications due to the health care intervention. The preponderance of evidence in outcome studies is that they reduce the risk of wrong-site surgery and overall morbidity and mortality associated with surgical care.[13] They also improve the cohesiveness of the surgical team and promote a culture of safety.

If the specialty needs convincing, The Checklist Manifesto, by Atul Gawande,[14] offers a strong case for promoting safety and diminishing surgical ineptitude. The complexity of the clinical tasks required to perform ambulatory oral and maxillofacial surgery have accelerated to the point where errors are inevitable. Systems are needed to eliminate wrong-site surgery. Gawande convinces readers that change to promote a culture of safety and improve patient outcomes is possible and necessary. It is time for the specialty of oral and maxillofacial surgery to incorporate its own customized national patient safety standards to improve patient outcomes. Incorporating checklists into oral and maxillofacial surgical practice will create special challenges but with enormous benefits.

REFERENCES

1. The joint commission ambulatory care patient safety goals. Available at: http://www.jointcommission.org/assets/1/6/2016_NPSG_AHC_ER.pdf. Accessed July 28, 2016.
2. Hughes RG. Patient Safety and quality: an evidence based handbook for nurses. Rockville (MD): Agency for Healthcare Resarch and quality; 2008.
3. Dental Anesthesia Assistant National Certification Examination. Rosemont (IL): American Association of Oral and Maxillofacial Surgeons; 2016. Available at: http://www.aaoms.org/continuing-education/certification-program-daance. Accessed August 21, 2016.
4. Smith R. Mark my tooth, patient safety network, agency for healthcare research and quality. US Dept of Health and Human Services. Available at: https://psnet.ahrq.gov/webmm/case/156/mark-my-tooth. Accessed August 1, 2016.
5. Lee JS, Curley JD, Smith RA. Prevention of worng site tooth extraction: clinical guidelines. J Oral Maxillofac Surg 2009;65(9):1793–9.
6. Kumar KK. Tooth Numbering System/tooth identification systems. Available at: http://www.slideshare.net/KishorKumar56/tooth-numbering-system. Accessed August 2, 2016.
7. Chang HH, Lee JJ, Cheng SH. Effectiveness of an educational program in reducing the incidence of wrong site tooth extraction. Oral Surg 2004;98:288–94.
8. Imai M. What is Kaizen. Tokyo: Kaizen Institute; 2016. Available at: https://www.kaizen.com/about-us/kaizen-institute.html. Accessed August 6, 2016.
9. Haynes AB, Weiser TG, Berry WR, et al, For the Safe Surgery Saves Lives Study Group. A surgical safety checklist to reduce morbidity and mortality in a global population. N Engl J Med 2009;360:491–9.
10. WHO guidelines for safe surgery 2009. Safe surgery saves lives. Available at: http://apps.who.int/iris/bitstream/10665/44185/1/9789241598552_eng.pdf. Accessed Auguest 7, 2016.
11. The WHO surgical safety checklist and implementation manual. Geneva (Switzerland): World Health Organization Press; 2016.
12. Surgical Safety Checklist WHO. Available at: http://www.who.int/patientsafety/safesurgery/tools_resources/SSSL_Checklist_finalJun08.pdf?ua=1. Accessed July 31, 2016.
13. Walker A, Resamwalla S, Wilson I. Surgical safety checklists: do they improve outcomes? Br J Anaesth 2012;109(1):47–54.
14. Gawande A. The checklist manifesto, how to get things right. New York: Holt Henry & Co; 2009.

Monitoring for the Oral and Maxillofacial Surgeon

Robert C. Bosack, DDS*

KEYWORDS

- Anesthesia monitoring • Capnography • Pulse oximetry • Electrocardiography
- Oscillometric blood pressure recording • Pretracheal auscultation

KEY POINTS

- Office-based sedation is a stochastic process; variability of patient responses leads to unpredictability in achieving and maintaining an appropriate level of sedation.
- Unintentional or unanticipated oversedation will lead to diminution of airway tone and ventilatory urge, both of which can lead to early hypoxemia if not rapidly identified.
- Level of consciousness, oxygenation, ventilation, and circulation (and temperature when appropriate) must be continuously monitored during the administration of anesthesia.
- Robust monitoring guides anesthetic drug titration and facilitates early identification and remediation of adversity.
- Inherent limitations in the information provided by various monitors reminds the clinician to continually use her or his senses of sight and sound to complement information provided by monitoring devices.

INTRODUCTION

The purpose of this article is to highlight commonly used monitoring modalities during the delivery of various levels of office-based, open airway anesthesia. Modes of action, interpretation, significance, and limitation of information obtained is reviewed. It is important to appreciate that this technology continually evolves, and that changes in "standards" or "guidelines" will naturally follow, albeit at nonuniform paces. The requirement of "evidence" to support changes in these documents has been questioned,[1,2] in view of the inability to design randomized, prospective, single-variable trials that potentially and unethically expose patients to noxious treatment or lack of treatment. In such instances, carefully contemplated "reason" must prevail, especially when there is a possibility of improving patient safety.

Centrally acting sedative, analgesic, hypnotic, and locally acting anesthetic drugs are administered in the oral and maxillofacial surgery office to diminish or eliminate discomfort, anxiety, memory, and awareness, and blunt the neuroendocrine stress response associated with surgical procedures. The rapid or slow onset of anticipated and unanticipated, positive and negative alterations in patient "status," involving depth of sedation/anesthesia, autonomic and cardiopulmonary systems, occur as a direct consequence of the challenges of surgery/sedation or a result of an adverse side effect or overdose of medications. These problems include oversedation,

The author has no disclosures or conflicts of interest to report.
College of Dentistry, University of Illinois at Chicago, 801 S Paulina Street, Chicago, IL 60612
* 16011 South 108th Avenue, Orland Park, IL 60467.
E-mail address: r.bosack@comcast.net

Oral Maxillofacial Surg Clin N Am 29 (2017) 159–168
http://dx.doi.org/10.1016/j.coms.2016.12.008
1042-3699/17/© 2016 Elsevier Inc. All rights reserved.

undersedation, exacerbation of underlying disease, aspiration, compromise or loss of upper airway tone and patency, diminished or eliminated ventilatory drive, predisposition to laryngospasm, increases or decreases in blood pressure and heart rate, and perturbation of heart rhythm, among others. As these problems are anticipated, "continual watchfulness" is mandated to facilitate early identification and remediation. Early identification will facilitate more rapid intervention, blunting the "time urgency," which may negatively affect performance. This is called *vigilance*, which is the motto of the American Society of Anesthesiologists.[3]

STANDARDS AND GUIDELINES

Although various agencies and organizations have difficulty in agreeing to a uniform "set of rules/regulations/guidelines" for the indications and necessity of various monitoring devices during the various levels of sedation, there is uniformity in recommendations that the patient's level of sedation (consciousness), oxygenation, ventilation, circulation, and temperature (during the use of potential triggers of malignant hyperthermia) be continually evaluated during the delivery of anesthetics agents.[4] It is not the intent of this article to trigger conformity, but rather to stimulate a perceived need for intense monitoring during

anesthesia as a primary means to improve patient safety, in spite of the lack of supportive evidence-based data.[1]

THE PURSUIT OF PATIENT SAFETY

The physiologic variables accompanying the various depths of sedation have been defined[5] (**Table 1**). Several concepts can be gleaned from this chart. All of these various levels are drug-induced and reversible. The use of the words "usually," "may," and "frequently" imply that the divisions between these various levels can be arbitrary and patient responses to drug administration are continuously variable, which can facilitate rapid, and possibly unexpected movement between levels of sedation. Levels of sedation also vary with surgical stimulation, variability of drug onset, and accumulation/redistribution from fat or muscle stores to central nervous system receptors. It is precisely for this reason that practitioners should be able to rescue their patients from 1 level deeper than intended. This rescue includes support and maintenance of airway patency, ventilation, and cardiovascular parameters necessary for perfusion of vital organs. It stands to reason that monitoring should therefore be appropriate for at least 1 level deeper than the intended level of sedation.

Table 1
Continuum of depth of sedation: definition of general anesthesia and levels of sedation and analgesia

	Minimum Sedation (Anxiolysis)	Moderate Sedation/ Analgesia (Conscious Sedation)	Deep Sedation/ Analgesia	General Anesthesia
Responsiveness	Normal response to verbal stimulation	Purposeful[a] response to verbal or tactile stimulation	Purposeful[a] response after repeated or painful stimulation	Unarousable
Airway	Unaffected	No intervention required	Intervention may be required	Intervention often required
Spontaneous ventilation	Unaffected	Adequate	May be inadequate	Frequently inadequate
Cardiovascular function	Unaffected	Usually maintained	Usually maintained	May be impaired

As sedation is a continuum, individual patient responses are variable and may not exactly follow these categorizations.
  [a] Reflex withdrawal from a painful stimulus is not considered a purposeful response.
  From American Society of Anesthesiologists. Continuum of depth of sedation: definition of general anesthesia and levels of sedation/analgesia. 1999. Last amended October 15, 2014. Available at: http://www.asahq.org/~/media/sites/asahq/files/public/resources/standards-guidelines/continuum-of-depth-of-sedation-definition-of-general-anesthesia-and-levels-of-sedation-analgesia.pdf. Accessed May 24, 2016. Reprinted with permission of the American Society of Anesthesiologists, 1061 American Lane, Schaumburg IL.

PARAMETERS AND MODALITIES OF ANESTHETIC MONITORING
Level of Consciousness

The patient's level of consciousness after drug administration can be assessed by *observing and listening* for the presence, absence, delay, and appropriateness of responses to verbal and tactile stimulation. Verbal stimuli include directives to open the mouth, take a deep breath, and so forth. Tactile stimuli include tapping the patient's shoulder or stimulation from local anesthetic injection. Stimuli such as sternal rubs or ear pinching are practices often considered inappropriate, but may, in fact, be life-saving when required to immediately "rescue" an apneic patient from a deeper than intended level of sedation. Patient movement, grimacing, or tears is often a sign of light or insufficient anesthesia, and may herald unintentional awareness with recall. It is important to note that postanesthetic recall of intraoperative awareness can occur in the absence of these signs.[6]

Oxygenation

The concentration of oxygen in the blood is indirectly measured with pulse oximetry and should not be estimated by observing the color of the patient's skin/mucosa.

Cyanosis is a blue/purple coloration most readily noted on superficial skin, nail beds, and mucous membranes when a concentration of 5 g/dL of reduced (deoxygenated) hemoglobin is reached. Anemic patients can be hypoxemic without cyanosis, whereas polycythemic patients can be cyanotic without hypoxemia. Cyanosis is less noticeable in patients with pigmented skin or in rooms with poor lighting. Peripheral vasoconstriction can cause nail beds to appear blue even when reduced hemoglobin is less than 5 g/dL. Cyanosis is an approximate, and at times, unreliable indicator of hypoxemia. Cyanosis has been reported to correspond to an SaO_2 (oxygen saturation of hemoglobin in arterial blood) of 67%.[7] If the patient becomes cyanotic, it is a late sign that should have been detected earlier by pulse oximetry. Monitoring oxygenation based solely on cyanosis is inappropriate.

Pulse oximetry
Pulse oximetry is a safe, convenient, noninvasive spectrophotometric modality that continuously measures the concentration of oxyhemoglobin in arterial blood (SpO_2). A finger probe is commonly used, which consists of 22 light-emitting diodes that emit different wavelengths of light. Based on the principle that oxygenated hemoglobin selectively absorbs more infrared (invisible) light (940 nm), whereas deoxygenated hemoglobin selectively absorbs more red (visible) light (660 nm), a photodetector on the other side of the probe measures light that has not been absorbed by intervening tissue and pulsatile blood. The information is converted into a percentage value, which approximates the concentration of oxygenated hemoglobin divided by the sum of oxygenation and deoxygenated hemoglobin. As discussed previously, the device also functions as a plethysmograph and is able to display the pulse rate. Information from pulse oximetry is displaced as a percent value; most combination monitors will also displace a pulse waveform (**Fig. 1**).

An understanding of the physiology of oxygen transport and delivery will improve interpretation of the SpO_2 (the % of hemoglobin saturated with oxygen, as measured by *pulse oximetry*). In the blood, oxygen exists in 3 states: (1) freely diffusible gas, (2) (in equilibrium with) oxygen dissolved in plasma, and (3) (in equilibrium with) oxygen bound to hemoglobin. As blood cannot carry enough dissolved oxygen to meet metabolic demands, hemoglobin acts as a temporary reservoir, capable of binding and releasing large amounts of oxygen. The red blood cell contains a large supply of hemoglobin molecules (2 alpha and 2 beta subunits), each capable of binding 4 oxygen molecules in a cooperative fashion: each successive binding of 1 molecule progressively increases the binding affinity of the next molecule, a concept termed progressive "cooperativity." In a reverse, but similar fashion, each subsequent offloading of an oxygen molecule lessens the affinity of the remaining molecules, enhancing their release. Hemoglobin binds (will become saturated with) oxygen when the ambient oxygen pressure is high (pulmonary

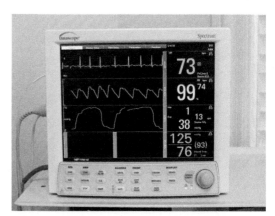

Fig. 1. Commonly used monitors during office-based anesthesia will simultaneously display waveforms of arterial pulsations and exhaled CO_2. (Mindray, Mahwah, NJ.)

alveoli) and releases oxygen when the ambient oxygen pressure is low (peripheral tissues). This relationship is graphically displayed in the oxygen-hemoglobin dissociation curve[8] (**Fig. 2**). Little change in hemoglobin saturation will occur at arterial oxygen tensions greater than 60 mm Hg, but when oxygen tension falls below 60 mm Hg, hemoglobin saturation rapidly plummets, triggering the so-called "time urgency" during airway rescue with hypoxia. As such, during the conduct of an anesthetic, even a 1% drop in SpO_2 should trigger an immediate and thorough evaluation of oxygen delivery to the lungs. For this reason, pulse oximetry has been termed "a sentry standing on the cliff of desaturation." As an additional safety measure, the pulse oximeter can be configured to audibly alarm at a threshold value, which would alert the entire team to potential airway or ventilatory demise. Based on the previous information, it would be prudent to set the alarm value somewhere between 90% and 95%, with 93% as a reasonable mean, to provide early warning, and yet avoid alarm fatigue.

There are several clinically significant limitations of pulse oximetry.

1. *Delayed detection of hemoglobin desaturation.* Signal averaging and circulation time from heart to probe delays detection of hypoxemia for 30 seconds or more. This is evidenced by a similar delay in improvement of SpO_2 after ventilatory rescue of an apneic and hypoxemic patient. Patient movement (light anesthesia, shivering, breathing) can introduce pulsations in venous blood that can decrease accuracy and further delay date. The Masimo oximeter uses technology that reduces false alarms due to movement.[9]

2. *Failure to detect hypoventilation/apnea during administration of supplemental oxygen.* Preoxygenation fills the functional residual capacity, which serves as a continual supply (reservoir) of oxygen in the event of apnea. In addition, oxygen can move (bulk flow and diffusion) past a patent upper airway and into the lungs of an apneic patient ("apneic oxygenation"), which, in some circumstances, can maintain hemoglobin saturation during apnea. Hypoventilation can go unnoticed, and hypercarbia may develop, possibly deepening the level of sedation.

3. *Environmental conditions causing spurious measurements.* Ambient light, improper probe placement, and electromagnetic radiation from nearby cell phones can interfere with oximetry.[10]

4. *Patient conditions causing spurious measurements.* Hypoperfusion at the site of measurement (hypotension, dysrhythmias, vasoconstriction) can yield a falsely low reading.

5. *Inability to differentiate dyshemoglobins.* Carboxyhemoglobin (recent tobacco smoke exposure) is falsely interpreted as oxyhemoglobin and can falsely elevate SpO_2 by 5% to 10%. Methemoglobin in concentrations greater than 1% also will yield false readings.[11] Interestingly, elevated glycohemoglobin also will falsely elevate readings.[12]

Pulse oximetry does not measure the actual concentration of delivered oxygen. If an advanced airway, such as a laryngeal mask airway or

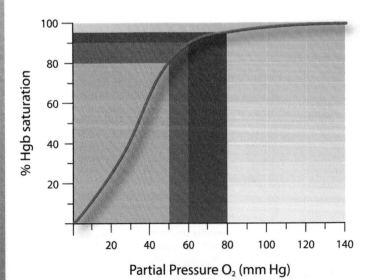

Fig. 2. The oxygen-hemoglobin dissociation curve. (*From* Bosack RC, Lee K. Limitations of patient monitoring during office-based anesthesia. In: Bosack RC, Lieblich S, editors. Anesthesia complications in the dental office. Ames (IA): Wiley Blackwell; 2014. p. 166; with permission.)

endotracheal tube is used, an oxygen gas analyzer connected directly to the breathing circuit must be used to ensure the delivery of a minimum concentration of 30% oxygen in the inspired gas.

Ventilation

Ventilation is the movement of gas to *and from* pulmonary alveoli. Gas movement is driven by pressure differences created by either negative pressure produced by bellows movement of the spontaneously ventilating patient or positive pressure from periodic compression of an airtight bag to push gas to the mouth (bag-valve-mask); larynx (laryngeal mask airway) or trachea (endotracheal tube). The movement of gas can be monitored by direct observation of chest excursions, periodic deflation of an oxygen reservoir bag, pretracheal auscultation, and capnography. A patient who is hiccupping, coughing, or speaking is, by definition, ventilating; however, even in these situations, there is still the possibility of inadequate gas exchange or respiratory distress.

Direct observation

Direct observation of rhythmic chest excursion is a somewhat crude method of ventilatory monitoring that is often not possible or reliable during surgical procedures, especially when patients are covered with baggy clothing and fluid-resistant bibs. In some instances, chest excursion can occur without ventilation. In such a circumstance, jerky "rocking boat" movement is noted when the chest paradoxically collapses and the abdomen protrudes during unsuccessful ventilatory attempts against a closed glottis (foreign body obstruction, laryngospasm). Sternal retraction can accompany these findings. Monitoring periodic deflation of a reservoir bag (not used with nasal cannulae) is also possible. Observation of ventilation will provide an indication of frequency, but will not provide reliable information of depth of ventilation.

Pretracheal auscultation

Pretracheal auscultation allows the clinician to listen to real-time sounds that accompany air movement throughout the respiratory tract.[13] Technology has significantly improved with the availability of Bluetooth wireless transmission to small earpieces, with which multiple clinicians can listen simultaneously (**Figs. 3** and **4**). Audible vibrations that occur with air movement behave in similar fashion to blood flow murmurs. Noise is audible when turbulence occurs, as with fast air movement through a small-diameter tube. As such, a slowly ventilating patient with a wide open (upper and lower) airway may not be heard. In all other circumstances, the clinician can hear

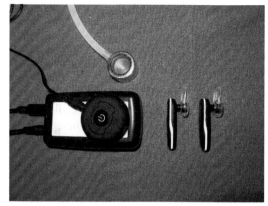

Fig. 3. Stethoscope with Bluetooth transmission to multiple earpieces.

impending airway collapse (supraglottic snoring), secretions near the larynx, early indications of laryngospasm (glottic crowing), or (subglottic) wheezing. A silent, bronchospastic chest also can be noted by total lack of breath sounds. Extraneous room noise (drilling, room ventilation, suction) will periodically interfere with auscultation. Auscultation informs little about depth of ventilation.

Capnography

Capnography refers to the time-oriented, continuous measurement of the concentration (partial pressure) of CO_2 in expired respiratory gases, with information revealed as both a number (capnogram) and a waveform (capnography). For CO_2 to appear in exhaled gas, 3 physiologic functions must be occurring: ongoing alveolar ventilation, diffusion of gas across the respiratory membrane, and adequate blood perfusion.

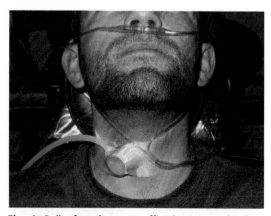

Fig. 4. Bell of stethoscope affixed to pretracheal region with circular double-sided adhesive tape, supported with surgical tape. Skin seal and sound quality is improved in the "para-tracheal" position.

Typically, a sidestream sample is aspirated through a 60-inch microbore tube by the monitor at a rate of approximately 150 mL/min, with concerns that higher rates contaminate the sample with ambient air and lower rates do not capture sufficient information. This distance accounts for an approximately 6-second delay in measurement. There are several sources of sampling error in open airway situations, depending on the location sampled. Nasal cannula sampling will fail in patients with nasal congestion or in instances of mouth breathing. If sampling occurs under a nasal hood, continual oxygen or oxygen/nitrous oxide mixtures will dilute exhaled gases, yielding low or absent readings. Because exhaled air is humidified, water condensation can obstruct the sampling line, or lead to falsely elevated readings.[14] For this reason, most capnographs will have water traps or filters. In most instances, end-tidal CO_2 measurements can be 5 to 10 mm Hg lower than the normal $Paco_2$ of 40 mm Hg, as breathing circuits are open and subject to room air dilution. CO_2 concentrations are measured via infrared spectrometry.

A typical CO_2 waveform is shown in **Fig. 5**. During the conduct of an office-based, open airway anesthetic, all team members can readily identify the humps that accompany exhalation. Decreases in both frequency and depth of ventilation are expected with the administration of opioids and hypnotics, and benzodiazepines, due to synergistic pharmacologic amplification of opioids and hypnotics. Of note, sudden loss of waveform, as depicted in **Fig. 6**, is troublesome and demands immediate attention. Laryngospasm or upper or lower airway obstruction may the triggering event. Blunting of the alpha angle occurs with prolonged expiration, typical of a decrease in airway diameter, seen in bronchospasm, displaying the typical "shark-fin" pattern (**Fig. 7**).

Accuracy and timeliness of information regarding ventilatory status is optimized when capnography is combined with pretracheal auscultation, as each has both limitations and advantages, as seen in (**Table 2**). Notice the potential difficulty in ensuring ventilation in a patient who breathes slowly and silently through the mouth (**Table 2**).

Colorimetric CO_2 detectors

Colorimetric CO_2 detectors consist of a piece of litmus paper that changes color from purple to yellow when exposed to greater than 15 mm Hg CO_2. Its use is to verify accurate placement of an endotracheal tube.

Circulation

Adequate blood pressure is necessary to perfuse all tissues with oxygen and glucose-enriched blood (circulation). As noted in **Fig. 8**, readily measurable parameters of circulation include blood pressure, heart rate, and heart rhythm.

During the conduct of an office-based anesthesia, blood pressures are typically measured every 5 minutes via *oscillometric pressure monitors*. In this instance, a cuff-inflation pump and bleed valve will pressurize a cuff typically applied to the upper arm to a pressure higher than systolic and then slowly release pressure to identify the beginning, maximal, and end of oscillations that occur with compression of the brachial artery. The point of maximal oscillations is the mean arterial pressure; from this value, systolic and diastolic are proprietarily measured.[15] Longer intervals between measurements can miss transient swings in pressure. These swings may be significant in elderly patients and in patients who are hypovolemic. In such cases, blood pressure measurement intervals can be shortened.

The width of the cuff should be approximately one-half the circumference of the arm. Loose or excessively large cuffs can underestimate pressure, whereas excessively tight or small cuffs can overestimate pressure. Cuffs should be placed at the level of the heart. Accuracy diminishes with dysrhythmia. Systolic pressure increases and diastolic pressure decreases as the cuff moves to the forearm.[15]

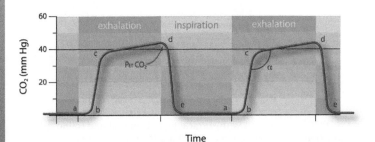

Fig. 5. A typical capnogram. (*From* Bosack RC, Lee K. Limitations of patient monitoring during office-based anesthesia. In: Bosack RC, Lieblich S, editors. Anesthesia complications in the dental office. Ames (IA): Wiley Blackwell; 2014. p. 167; with permission.)

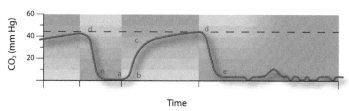

Fig. 6. Sudden loss of waveform. (*From* Bosack RC, Lee K. Limitations of patient monitoring during office-based anesthesia. In: Bosack RC, Lieblich S, editors. Anesthesia complications in the dental office. Ames (IA): Wiley Blackwell; 2014. p. 167; with permission.)

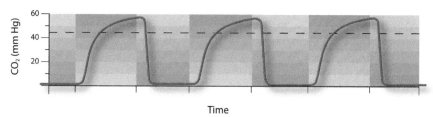

Fig. 7. Shark-fin capnographic tracing, as seen in bronchospasm. (*From* Bosack RC, Lee K. Limitations of patient monitoring during office-based anesthesia. In: Bosack RC, Lieblich S, editors. Anesthesia complications in the dental office. Ames (IA): Wiley Blackwell; 2014. p. 167; with permission.)

Table 2
Comparative sensitivity of capnography and pretracheal auscultation in various clinical scenarios

	Side Stream, Nasal Sampling Capnography	Pretracheal Auscultation
Mouth breather	No	Yes
Slow, silent nasal breathing	Yes	No
Slow, silent mouth breathing	No	No
Able to detect impending airway compromise	No	Yes
Able to detect wheezing	No	Yes

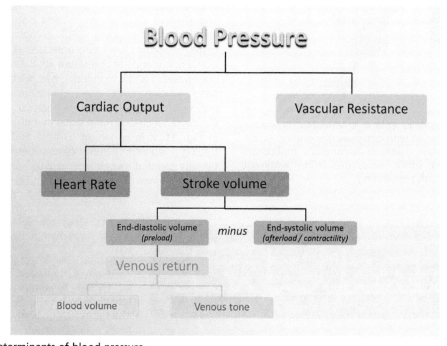

Fig. 8. Determinants of blood pressure.

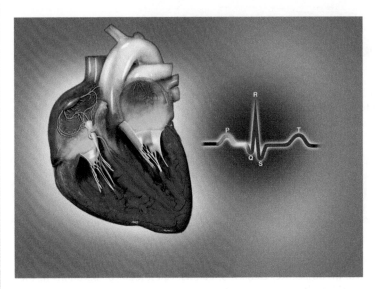

Fig. 9. Spatial progression of electrical potentials of the heart, with sequential contribution to the classic ECG tracing. (*From* Anderson E, Bosack R. Anesthetic considerations for patients with cardiovascular disease. In: Bosack RC, Lieblich S, editors. Anesthesia complications in the dental office. Ames (IA): Wiley Blackwell; 2014. p. 35; with permission.)

HEART RATE AND RHYTHM

As outlined in **Fig. 8**, heart rate (rhythm) is one determinant of cardiac output, which in turn affects blood pressure. *Electrocardiography* (ECG) is the amplified surface recording of the sum of all electrical potentials generated by depolarization of myocytes, displayed as a continuous waveform (**Fig. 9**). A lead II tracing (**Figs. 10** and **11**) is routinely used in the office, as this vector best aligns with the net movement of depolarization. In most instances of lead II waveforms, P waves and P-wave changes are clearly displayed, followed by an upgoing QRS complex. Benign rhythm disorders are easily noted, as is the occasional occurrence of premature atrial or ventricular complexes. Lead II monitoring has not been identified as being sensitive to irregularities in repolarization or predictive of myocardial ischemia. Characteristics of normal sinus rhythm are shown in **Fig. 11**. It is important to note that the ECG tracing gives information only about electrical potentials and that myocyte contraction occurs after the appearance of depolarization and is verified by

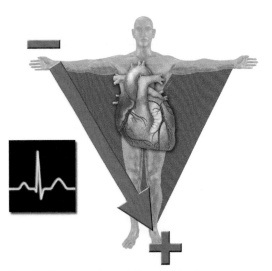

Fig. 10. Configuration of limb electrodes for lead II. (*From* Anderson E, Bosack R. Anesthetic considerations for patients with cardiovascular disease. In: Bosack RC, Lieblich S, editors. Anesthesia complications in the dental office. Ames (IA): Wiley Blackwell; 2014. p. 36; with permission.)

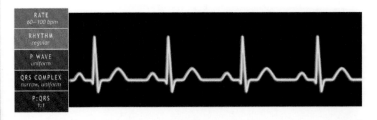

Fig. 11. Characteristics of lead II normal sinus rhythm. (*From* Anderson E, Bosack R. Anesthetic considerations for patients with cardiovascular disease. In: Bosack RC, Lieblich S, editors. Anesthesia complications in the dental office. Ames (IA): Wiley Blackwell; 2014. p. 35; with permission.)

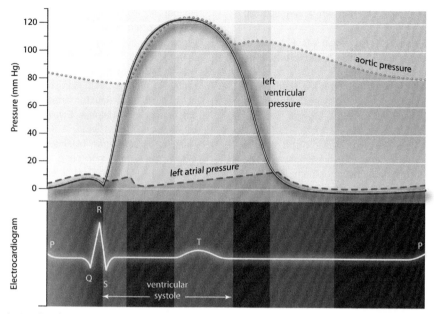

Fig. 12. Relationship between the ECG and myocyte contraction/pressure generation.

pulse oximetry and blood pressure, as shown in **Fig. 12.**

It is important to be mindful of the relationship between the ECG, which provides information about electrical potentials, and myocyte contraction, which occurs after the appearance of depolarization and leads to the development of the pressure that drives blood flow in the circulatory system, verified by pulse oximetry and blood pressure measurement. A summary redrawing of the classic Wiggers diagram visually depicts this relationship (**Fig. 12**).

SUMMARY

From the foregoing, it becomes apparent that the clinician must be vigilant to a host of physiologic parameters, and that no one monitor is able to "tell the whole story." Each modality (direct visualization, SpO₂, capnography, pretracheal auscultation, and ECG [rate and rhythm]), when used in concert with all others will give the most complete and timely picture of the patient's status during the administration of anesthetic agents. The concept of the anesthetic team, with formal training of anesthesia assistants, is emphasized.

REFERENCES

1. Leape LL, Berwick DM, Bates DW. What practices will most improve safety? Evidence-based medicine meets patient safety. JAMA 2002;288:501–7.
2. Shelley K. Noninvasive hemodynamic monitoring. ASA Monitor 2011;75:18–9.
3. Bacon DR. Iconography in anesthesiology. The importance of society seals in the 1920s and 30s. Anesthesiology 1996;85:414–9.
4. American Society of Anesthesiologists. Standards for basic anesthesia monitoring. 1986. Amended October 20, 2010. Affirmed October 28, 2015. Available at: http://www.asahq.org/~/media/sites/asahq/files/public/resources/standards-guidelines/standards-for-basic-anesthetic-monitoring.pdf. Accessed May 24, 2016.
5. American Society of Anesthesiologists. Continuum of depth of sedation: definition of general anesthesia and levels of sedation/analgesia. 1999. Last amended October 15, 2014. Available at: http://www.asahq.org/~/media/sites/asahq/files/public/resources/standards-guidelines/continuum-of-depth-of-sedation-definition-of-general-anesthesia-and-levels-of-sedation-analgesia.pdf. Accessed May 24, 2016.
6. Bosack RC. Post-anesthetic recall of intraoperative awareness. In: Bosack RC, Lieblich S, editors. Anesthesia complications in the dental office. Ames (IA): Wiley Blackwell; 2014. p. 283–5.
7. Grace RF. Pulse oximetry: gold standard or false sense of security? Med J Aust 1994;260:638–44.
8. Bosack RC, Lee K. Limitations of patient monitoring during office-based anesthesia. In: Bosack RC, Lieblich S, editors. Anesthesia complications in the dental office. Ames (IA): Wiley Blackwell; 2014. p. 163–9.
9. Malviya S, Reynolds PI, Voepel-Lewis T, et al. False alarms and sensitivity of conventional pulse oximetry versus the Masimo SET technology in pediatric

postanesthesia care unit. Anesth Analg 2000;90: 1336–40.

10. Ralston AC, Webb RK, Runciman WB. Potential errors in pulse oximetry. I. Pulse oximeter evaluation. Anaesthesia 1991;46:202–6.

11. Torp KD. Pulse oximetry. In: Murray MJ, Harrison BA, Mueller JT, et al, editors. Faust's anesthesiology review. 4th edition. Philadelphia: Elsevier Sanders; 2015. p. 31–2.

12. Pu LJ, Shen Y, Lu L, et al. Increased blood glycohemoglobin A1c levels lead to overestimation of arterial oxygen saturation by pulse oximetry in patients with type 2 diabetes. Cardiovasc Diabetol 2012;11: 110–5.

13. Boriosi JP, Hollman GA. Making a case for use of the pretracheal stethoscope in pediatric procedural sedation. Pediatr Anesth 2016;26: 249–55.

14. Ivancic MG. Carbon dioxide retention and capnography. In: Murray MJ, Harrison BA, Mueller JT, et al, editors. Faust's anesthesiology review. 4th edition. Philadelphia: Elsevier Sanders; 2015. p. 17–9.

15. Humpherys CG, Murray MJ. Intermittent noninvasive blood pressure monitoring. In: Murray MJ, Harrison BA, Mueller JT, et al, editors. Faust's anesthesiology review. 4th edition. Philadelphia: Elsevier Sanders; 2015. p. 37–40.

Simulation Training for the Office-Based Anesthesia Team

Richard M. Ritt, EMT-P, MA[a],*, Jeffrey D. Bennett, DMD[b],
David W. Todd, DMD, MD, FACD[c]

KEYWORDS

- Team • Staff • Simulation • Training • Emergency • Office roles

KEY POINTS

- In the event of a medical emergency or crisis, a successful patient outcome relies on how well the office staff work together as a team.
- It is imperative to have a means to organize and optimize the resources of the entire office to provide the best possible care in case of an emergency.
- A pragmatic hands-on team training approach for in situ dental emergencies using simulation should be used.
- The future of simulation will involve 3 different models of simulation to address cost effectiveness and clinical applications: physical reality (patient mannequins), screen-based simulation, and virtual reality with either 2-D or 3-D with or without physical tools.
- Further research is needed to clarify how to most effectively use simulation to learn and maintain clinical proficiency in both routine and rarely used emergency situations.

INTRODUCTION

An OMS office is a complex environment. Within such an environment, a diverse scope of complex surgical procedures is performed with different levels of anesthesia, ranging from local anesthesia to general anesthesia, on patients with varying comorbidities. Optimal patient outcomes require a functional surgical and anesthetic team, who are familiar with both standard operational principles and emergency recognition and management. Offices with high volume and time pressure add further stress and potential risk to the office environment. Creating and maintaining a functional surgical and anesthetic team that is competent with a culture of patient safety and risk reduction is a significant challenge that requires time, commitment, planning, and

dedication. This article focuses on the role of simulation training in office training and preparation.

WHAT IS SIMULATION?

Medical simulation is an artificial representation or imitation of a real event or process. It provides a safe environment, often immersive in nature, for both doctor and staff to have unlimited exposure to various experiences, both routine treatment and infrequent emergencies, without adverse consequences to any patient (**Box 1**). It is beneficial in providing education and assessment of both individual and team performance and of system operation and functionality. Both the educational and assessment components of simulation training are essential to simulation training. The simulation experience is actually incomplete without the

Disclosures: None.
[a] Consultant Dental Simulation Specialists Inc, 22721 Foxtail Drive, Kildeer, IL 60047, USA; [b] 1481 West 10th Street, Indianapolis, IN 46202, USA; [c] Private Practice, 120 Southwestern Drive, Lakewood, NY 14750, USA
* Corresponding author.
E-mail address: Dentalsimulationspecialists@gmail.com

Oral Maxillofacial Surg Clin N Am 29 (2017) 169–178
http://dx.doi.org/10.1016/j.coms.2016.12.006
1042-3699/17/© 2017 Elsevier Inc. All rights reserved.

Box 1
Advantages of simulation training

1. Provide education and assessment in clinical operation (both routine and emergent)
2. Repetitive practice to address performance gaps without putting patients at risk
3. Real time "deliberate" practice of infrequent medical emergencies
4. Standardized experience with most emergency scenarios
5. Safe environment for both the doctor and staff members
6. Team and crisis resource training that is specific to the environment and personnel
7. Unlimited exposure to high-risk, low-incident cases
8. Ability to organize and customize training opportunities
9. Ability to provide immediate feedback
10. Opportunity for the entire office team to participate in training[13]

---

assessment or debriefing session. The debriefing provides an opportunity for the team to reflect on their performance in which strengths, weaknesses, and gaps are identified, which allows for an office to optimize operations, enhance dental team performance, and ultimately improve patient outcomes.

Simulation training develops both the individual and the team. Individual development focuses on knowledge, task acquisition, and equipment and drug familiarity. Team development emphasizes leadership, role delegation, workload distribution, closed loop communication, staff member empowerment, documentation, and stress reduction.

THE NEED FOR OFFICE-BASED SIMULATION TRAINING

In the hospital, there is a team of internal medical doctors, anesthesiologists, medical specialists, nurses, respiratory therapists, and pharmacists, who can respond to a medical challenge or medical emergency. By the simple nature of the hospital environment, this team is regularly exposed to complex medical situations. Even though medical emergency intervention is routine for this team of highly trained medical staff, many hospitals have regularly scheduled simulated drills throughout the hospital for certain scenarios.

In an OMS office, the minimal staffing may consist of 1 doctor, 1 anesthetic assistant, 1 surgical assistant, and possibly 1 front office staff member. Although many states require Advanced Cardiac Life Support (ACLS) and Pediatric Advanced Life Support (PALS) for anesthesia certificates and the Office Anesthesia Evaluation program recommends regular emergency drills, there may be no mandatory training for anesthetic and surgical assistants other than Basic Life Support (BLS). This environment necessitates a different team model. Additionally, an OMS office is not a critical care center and the office may never or infrequently have been involved in the management of a medical challenge or medical emergency.

TYPES OF SIMULATORS

There are a variety of simulators that can be used to improve methods/processes (**Box 2**) and skills (**Box 3**) for managing both routine care and office emergencies. Simple task trainers have been shown to teach skills that transfer well to clinical care. Simple airway manikins allow bag-valve-mask (BVM) ventilation, nasopharyngeal and oral airway placement, supraglottic airway placement, and endotracheal intubation. By definition, most of the task simulators used in BLS and ACLS are simple simulators that do not expose a trainee to complex and difficult airway management tasks and scenarios. Cardiopulmonary resuscitation (CPR) manikins can be low fidelity with compression practice or high fidelity with recording of tidal volume, respiratory rate, compression depth, and compression rate. Simulation can be software based, where participants respond to a vital signs monitor display and manipulate tasks and drugs according to options in the menu. These programs can be used

---

Box 2
Procedural processes

1. Patient triage
   a. Taking and documenting vital signs
   b. How to review medical history
   c. Recognizing subtle signs of medical conditions
   d. Preanesthetic questions
2. Checklist
3. Timeout
4. Communication (closed loop)
5. Teamwork
6. Equipment familiarity
7. Drug familiarity
8. Intraoperative monitoring
9. Postoperative monitoring
10. Discharge operation

Box 3
Tasks/skills

1. Airway management

   a. How to set up airway equipment and instrumentation

   b. How to use an oxygen tank

   c. How to place a nasal cannula

   d. How to place a nasopharyngeal or oropharygngeal airway

   e. Mask ventilation

   f. Supraglottic airway/endotracheal tube placement

2. Vascular access

   a. How to set up IV equipment

   b. Choosing intravascular fluid

   c. How to set the flow of an IV line

   d. How to secure an IV line

   e. How to run an infusion pump

   f. How to set up intraosseous access

3. Drug preparation

   a. Identify drug (many drugs have similar names or come in similar packages; a step to minimize drug confusion is to limit concentrations of the same drug and to avoid drugs with similar packaging)

   b. How to open an ampule

   c. How to draw up a drug from a sealed vial

   d. How to label a syringe

   e. How to dilute a drug and prepare the necessary concentration and dose

4. Drug administration

   a. How to administer an IV drug

   b. Closed loop communication

      1. You want drug name followed by drug dosage administered IV now

      2. I have administered drug name followed by drug dosage now

   c. How to flush the line after drug administration

5. Defibrillator/cardioversion/pacer

   a. Know how to set up machine and pad placement

   b. Know proper management of sync versus unsync energy delivery

   c. Know correct energy levels

---

by practitioners to refine clinical knowledge or by office staff to demonstrate basic concepts, role responsibility, and team function. The highest level of simulation provides an artificial replication of the clinical setting, which fully immerses a team into an experience that simulates both routine operation and emergency scenarios. This can involve human simulated patients (biological simulation) or high-fidelity simulation manikins. High-fidelity simulation manikins, such as the SimMan (Laerdal Medical Corporation, Wappingers Falls, NY), allow for airway interventions, intravenous (IV) fluid administration, CPR, defibrillation, and so forth.

This level of human simulation is unparalleled in that it provides an opportunity for practitioners to work with their own personnel, potentially within their own office environment, to address both routine operation and emergency scenarios.

WHAT IS LEARNED FROM EMERGENCY DRILLS?
Procedural Familiarity, Task Acquisition, and Assessment

Patient selection and anticipation and preparation for medical challenges and medical emergencies are the responsibility of an office and can both reduce adverse events and optimize patient outcome. Although this article is not focused on patient selection, a well-trained, empowered office staff may have a critical role in patient selection. Patients or patient escorts may share information with office staff that they may not share with the doctor. Office staff who accompany a patient into the operatory may recognize subtleties as patients walk down a hallway and enter a room that may not be obvious to a doctor whose encounter with patients is while they are seated in a surgical chair. A trained office staff member may not necessarily make a diagnosis but may be more likely to identify an abnormality or a deviation from "normal." A hierarchal environment that does not empower staff to fully contribute to patient care may miss this critical information.

Team empowerment is also critical and can optimize teamwork during an emergency. Every staff member should feel comfortable with communicating thoughts pertaining to patient assessment and intervention. An empowered staff who can inform a doctor of something that the doctor or more senior team member may not have recognized or may not be performing adequately may improve patient outcome. Alternatively, a lack of such communication can contribute to or worsen the outcome of an adverse outcome.

Current residents and practitioners who provide care in the hospital and The Joint Commission or comparably accredited offices are familiar with processes, such as checklists and timeout (see: Leon A. Assael, article "Preventing Wrong-Site Surgery in Oral and Maxillofacial Surgery," in this issue). These procedural processes are important and reduce adverse events. It is time for these processes to be incorporated into all OMS offices. The introduction of these changes is intended to be beneficial for patient care. Incorporating change into an office alters workflow, however, which can be associated with mental and physical demand that may have an impact on performance and effort and result in frustration. Using simulation as a component of office training allows for a smoother transition in which resource assessment can be accomplished to minimize overwhelming the system. Simulation can also ensure optimal system operation. Simulation centers that replicate hospital wards have all levels of staff, from clerical to clinical, participate in simulated experiences that reproduce basic procedures. An OMS office can achieve the same with simulating concepts, such as patient triage, timeout, checklists, and so forth.

There are multiple tasks that are required for both routine care and emergency care (see **Box 3**). An area of focus is on airway management

because many of the most common serious complications and emergencies experienced in office-based anesthetic practice are related to airway management. Approximately 90% of airway emergencies can be corrected with simple measures, such as airway repositioning, nasopharyngeal or oropharyngeal airway placement, and effective BVM ventilation. All OMS staff are required to successfully participate in BLS biannually. The airway challenge and the level of acquired skill provided by BLS, however, do not equate to the clinical environment during ambulatory anesthesia, especially a difficult and challenging patient airway. The first time taking a mannequin-acquired airway skill to a real clinical environment, even one in which conditions are optimal, may result in a less than 50% success.[1] Furthermore, these skills can deteriorate over time without practice, and an exposure every 2 years does not amount to a well-trained office. All OMSs administering office-based anesthesia are required to successfully participate in ACLS biannually. Likewise neither does the airway challenge equate to the difficult airway nor is the time-limited recertification course sufficient to maintain skill and/or knowledge of emergency management without repeated re-exposure throughout the year. Some offices in which general anesthesia is performed have both surgeon and office staff perform BVM ventilation on patients during the procedure so that the process is not novel when required during an emergency. Task simulators attempt to replicate a real patient and enable staff to learn new skills and practice these skills.

Although most emergencies requiring ventilation can be managed with BVM ventilation, there are situations in which intubation may be advantageous or required. Direct laryngoscopy has traditionally been used to facilitate airway intubation but at times may be unsuccessful. Videolaryngoscopy, for most anesthesiologists, is becoming the most commonly used technique to rescue failed direct laryngoscopy and in some situations is replacing direct laryngoscopy as the instrument to initially achieve intubation.[2] Practicing OMSs, except for those recently graduated, most likely have not been exposed to videolaryngoscopy, which has become integrated into anesthetic care as standard equipment. Task simulators, therefore, provide an environment in which a practicing OMS may achieve a level of familiarity with a device, which should probably be a component of the emergency instrumentation. Furthermore, studies have demonstrated OMSs removed from residency training to be able to demonstrate satisfactory clinical use of the videolaryngoscope with task simulators.[3]

A new facility is an exciting time for a practice yet potentially hides unrecognized and latent threats to patient safety. These threats may be secondary to missing or inappropriately placed equipment, deficient system operation, disorganized office layout, unfamiliarity with the new office environment, or insufficient space. A simulated drill has the potential to identify the errors that may occur during a real-time event and allow for potential threats to be corrected. As important as it is to involve all office staff in the simulation exercise, there is also benefit to getting to know and inviting the local emergency response staff to participate in these exercises when opening a new facility, when a new doctor joins an office, or as the emergency response staff change. This orientation allows an OMS office staff to share the emergency plan with the emergency response staff, which may include how best the emergency response staff can enter and maneuver their stretcher in the facility. Alternatively, the emergency response staff may identify aspects of an emergency plan that are problematic and not recognized by office staff and offer alternate suggestions or improvements. Additionally, facilitating transfer of care can optimize patient care, and the emergency response staff can share with office staff what information they would appreciate being available on their arrival.

There are advances in knowledge and technology, and surgeons introduce new procedures into offices throughout their professional careers. The goal is to expand the services of an office and optimize patient care. Although these procedural changes are intended to improve office function and optimize patient care, there may be unrecognized and unanticipated consequences resulting in adverse outcomes. Having an office staff simulate the new methods or techniques prior to implementation on a patient may identify errors or problems with procedural modifications that allow for correction before an adverse patient occurrence.

Team Function

Knowledge maintenance and keeping abreast of current concepts, such as reading the literature or attending lectures at a medical conference, are common methods of continuing education, which are frequently done individually. Yet care is delivered is by a team. Optimal outcome depends on the functionality of a team.

A trained anesthetic assistant can improve quality of patient care and reduce both the quantity of errors and the severity of the errors for the potential harm they may cause.[4,5] The American Association of Oral and Maxillofacial Surgeons has developed the Dental Anesthesia Assistant National Certification Examination program to develop trained anesthetic assistants. This course may provide a foundation on which to begin. It is limited, however, in exposing participants to difficult and challenging procedures and tasks, which are critical to patient outcome. Participation and completion of the course is mandated neither by most state laws nor by a professional association. There is no documentation as to the effect it has in optimizing the delivery of care or reducing adverse events. Additionally, if the certification program is mandated, office staff turnover, especially, in small offices, may present difficulty with an office's ability to maintain compliance. The importance of a trained assistant, however, is especially critical in a small office with 1 practitioner, in which the doctor during an emergency finds himself or herself assessing a patient, being team lead, and performing many if not all major tasks and procedures because the staff is inadequately trained.

With a doctor being both team leader and the primary individual performing tasks, there is the potential to become fixated on a specific task. Crew resource management (CRM) principles for a hospital code recommend that the sole doctor, as team leader, position himself or herself in a position to observe and direct and allow the nursing, respiratory, and pharmacy staff be relegated to performing the tasks. Most OMS offices do not employ professionals, such as nurses or pharmacists. This concept is, therefore, difficult to replicate, emphasizing the importance of having a trained staff and the importance of preparation through simulation. Training provides a better understanding of roles, sharing of information, fostering interprofessional communication and collaboration, and a comfort and familiarity with each other in addition to improved skills and task capabilities (**Box 4**).

CRITICAL CARE PATHWAYS AND EMERGENCY MANUALS

Airway obstruction, hypoventilation, and oxygen desaturation are representations of potential problems that may occur during an anesthetic. Continuous observation and monitoring, airway positioning or repositioning, suctioning, and anesthetic drug titration are tasks routinely performed throughout the delivery of an anesthetic. For a well-trained individual and team, the subtleties in a patient's physiologic status are unconsciously recognized, communicated, and addressed individually and collectively. The process is frequently mundane, consisting of the same repetitive steps;

> **Box 4**
> **Goals of simulation**
>
> 1. Knowledge reinforcement
> 2. Leadership
> 3. Team training
> 4. Staff member empowerment
> 5. Workload distribution
> 6. Role delegation
> 7. Closed loop communication
> 8. Skill acquisition
> 9. Equipment/drug familiarity
> 10. Documentation
> 11. Patient disposition
> 12. Stress inoculation training

organized and cohesive response that efficiently uses the staff who are present at that time, which may vary by day.

Preassigned roles and responsibilities of staff promote a more efficient and organized team approach to managing a medical emergency. Emergency tasks and responsibilities are identified in **Box 5**. A representation of task delineation in an office with 1 doctor and 3 staff (anesthesia assistant, surgical assistant, and front-desk clerk) is provided in **Table 1**. There is no evidence, however, to suggest that the assistant airway training that is currently accepted as standard of care is sufficient, such that most assistants should be independently capable of managing the emergent airway. Although there is a lack of literature pertaining to the OMS model, the emergency and simulation literature suggest that more training is required to achieve an acceptable degree of success. State law may further compound emergency management, which limits who can prepare and administer medication.

but when the process is followed, patient care most frequently is uneventful.

Best practice is achieved through the establishment of structured protocol. Clinical care pathways optimize patient care and reduce negative outcome. They are important for both routine and emergency situations. Emergency and checklist manuals are used in many high-hazard industries. During a high-stress emergency situation, especially when such situations are rare, even the best of medical personal and teams may have an inability to retrieve knowledge from long-term memory that is rarely used.[6] The high stress of the emergent and unanticipated event may also contribute to an increase in omitting known steps.[7] Emergency manuals consisting of a context-relevant set of cognitive aids and checklists simplify and enable emergency medical intervention.[8,9] An example of such a cognitive aid is the "Emergency Therapy for Malignant Hyperthermia"[10] procedural poster that hangs in many hospital operating rooms.

ROLES AND RESPONSIBILITIES

Oral surgery facilities differ in size, type, number of staff, and overall organization of the office environment. Routinely, personnel included in providing sedation in the operatory consist of the doctor, surgical assistant, and anesthesia assistant; and in some offices there may be a fourth assistant. Depending on office size, there are a variety of front office staff and additional surgical staff. A multidoctor office may have more than 1 surgeon available. Regardless of office size, when an office crisis or emergency arises, there needs to be an

DOES SIMULATION MAKE A DIFFERENCE?

Participants favorably perceive simulation training as an education method. Task simulators have demonstrated effectiveness to achieve a level of skill for various procedures, which is transferable to clinical practice. Additionally, simulation-based

> **Box 5**
> **Emergency tasks and responsibilities**
>
> 1. Team leader
> 2. Procure emergency cart/kit
> 3. Read emergency manual — checklist
> 4. Airway management
> 5. Monitor — take vital signs
> 6. Interpret ECG
> 7. IV insertion
> 8. Drug preparation
> 9. Drug administration
> 10. Chest compressions
> 11. Defibrillator use
> 12. Documentation
> 13. Call for emergency assistance
> 14. Meet and direct EMS
> 15. Manage waiting room/interact with escort
> 16. Prepare records for transfer to EMS

Table 1
Task delineation for office staff

Doctor	Anesthesia Assistant	Surgical Assistant	Front-Office Clerk
Team oversight	Airway management	Procuring emergency cart	Reads emergency manual/checklist
Establishes diagnosis and activates emergency	Monitor	Drug preparation*	Documents
	Interprets ECG	Drug administration*	Calls 911
Requests emergency instrumentation	Assesses vital signs	IV set-up preparation*	Manages waiting room
	Alerts doctor to changes in vital signs	Chest compressions	Interacts with patient escort
Airway management	Obtains vital signs	Defibrillator use	Meets and direct EMS
Interprets ECG			Prepare records for transfer to EMS
Interprets vital signs			
Drug preparation*			
Drug administration*			
IV insertion*			
Chest compressions			
Defibrillator use			
Decision to activate 911			

* Task delineation may be limited by state law.

education can improve performance and adherence to emergency protocol and processes that are transferable to clinical practice. Simulation-based training compared with non–simulation-based training demonstrated better knowledge and skill retention. The evidence suggests, however, that the gain in knowledge and skills diminishes with time without reinforcement and repetitive training.

There are no studies to suggest the benefit of anesthesia and medical emergency simulation training in OMS practice. This is important because OMS practice differs from specialty practices, such as emergency medicine, anesthesiology, internal medicine, and others, that are hospital based. These practitioners are immersed into an environment in which they may frequently be challenged to use the knowledge and skill acquired in the simulation training. Experience is important, but simulation training has further benefit because, when comparing individuals with comparable experience, the individual who was provided simulation training demonstrated a higher level of performance.[11]

Whether high-fidelity simulations offer better educational outcomes versus more simple skills trainers or whether simulation offers better education compared with traditional lecture format depends on which outcomes are measured. Generally, in terms of knowledge transfer, simulation is equal to or slightly better than nonsimulation activities. In terms of skills transfer, simulation is more effective than nonsimulation activities. In terms of teaching nontechnical skills, such as CRM, simulation training is less well proved and harder to assess

in terms of benefit. In terms of generalization to clinical care and improved outcomes, except for specific treatment protocols in the delivery room (shoulder dystocia) and the emergency room (CPR and local anesthetic systemic toxicity response), simulation training has yet to prove its benefit. In addition, more study is needed to reflect on simulation training on initial learning versus long-term skill retention and clinical outcomes.

The frequency of a significant morbidity or mortality in an individual office is low. This makes it difficult to assess the effectiveness of simulation training on modifying quality of care and outcomes. Additionally, the low occurrence of morbidity and mortality as reported by OMS National Insurance Company, which is further supported by the literature, suggests that practicing OMSs lack current real-life experience in managing anesthetic and medical emergencies. The effectiveness of simulation training and regular mock exercises can, therefore, only be assessed by performance on simulation exercises and less likely by changes in patient care or outcomes. This is generally true for simulation training in general where improved patient outcomes across hospital systems or patient care groups is hard to demonstrate.

The American Association of Oral and Maxillofacial Surgeons recommends that the doctors and staff in OMS offices partake in periodic scheduled emergency management practice sessions, with which the authors concur.[12] The authors confer that simulation has the same benefit for OMS practice as is demonstrated in other realms. Additionally, because OMS practices are not routinely challenged with medical and anesthetic emergencies, practitioner and staff lack the added effect of experience on simulation training. Although there is no supportive evidence, it could be anticipated that this has an impact on retention of knowledge and skill resulting in a more rapid deterioration of capabilities. This further emphasizes the importance of frequent periodic emergency management practice sessions.

SIMULATION TRAINING SCENARIOS AND RESOURCES

It is vital that an entire team participate in the emergency exercises. Emergency drills should simulate both the common and rare emergency (**Box 6**). Offices should not only anticipate the rare emergency (eg, malignant hyperthermia) but the unusual and potentially complicating scenario (eg, mother faints, falls to ground, and bangs her head during induction of a 6-year-old child, and the office must maintain care of a sedated 6-year-old child and an unconscious mother with potential head trauma; or, a disruptive family member becomes aggressive during the medical management of a family member). The broad use of patient simulation as an educational activity prepares providers to:

- Focus on patient safety
- Practice high-risk, low-frequency cases
- Prepare for the what if and the unexpected
- Allow for repeated and deliberate practice
- Assume that one does best what one does most often[13]

Prior to a simulated case, it is helpful that an OMS team call a time-out in an effort to review and identify any potential precautions, complications, or concerns.

The most common errors observed in situ and in conference-sponsored simulations include a lack of closed-loop communication, missing or incomplete documentation, and inaccurate verification and administration of medications. There are several resources that are helpful when addressing communication issues, the need for continuous patient assessment, and maximizing personnel and other pertinent resources. Practicing the principles of CRM is another benefit of simulation training. Developed in response to airline disasters in the late 1980s, CRM principles allow for effective teamwork in times of emergency. The 6 goals of CRM are enhanced situational awareness, self-awareness, leadership, assertiveness, decision making, and communication. In 2011, the American Heart Association developed elements for team dynamics. These

| **Box 6** |
| **Office urgencies and emergencies** |

1. Cardiovascular
   a. Angina
   b. Myocardial infarction
   c. Cardiac arrest
   d. Hypotension
   e. Hypertension
   f. Bradycardia
   g. Tachycardia
   h. Dysrhythmia
2. Respiratory distress
   a. Hypoventilation
   b. Apnea
   c. Hyperventilation
   d. Oxygen desaturation
   e. Laryngospasm
   f. Bronchospasm
   g. Aspiration
   h. Airway obstruction (eg, foreign body or anaphylaxis)
3. Metabolic
   a. Hypoglycemia
   b. Hyperglycemia
4. Neurologic
   a. Seizure
   b. Altered mental status
   c. Loss of consciousness
   d. Agitation
   e. Psychiatric event
5. Disruptive escort
6. Nausea and vomiting
7. Malignant hyperthermia

elements emphasize the importance of closed-loop communication, clear roles and responsibilities, knowledge sharing, constructive intervention, and re-evaluation within an environment that fosters mutual respect and collegiality.[14–16] The Agency for Healthcare Research and Quality (2015) describes a TeamSTEPPS[17] approach that focuses on leadership, situation monitoring, mutual support, and communication. This approach empowers OMSs teams to resolve conflicts, practice routine and ongoing dialogue during all phases of patient care, and promote good teamwork. Last, the use of Plan-Do-Study-Act can also foster an overall commitment to continual examination and re-evaluation of each medical emergency or crisis for potential improvement opportunities.[18]

SHOULD THIS BE STANDARD OF CARE?

There is no substitute for periodic simulation training for medical emergencies and crisis in oral surgery offices. The opportunity to practice in an office with staff and equipment maximizes the hands-on learning experience. There are a variety of simulators and task trainers available that can be purchased or rented to conduct comprehensive and timely training in the dental practice. Staff members can engage in role play as the simulator and encourage discussion on a wide range of topics and scenarios. Other options include obtaining outside support that provides the simulation training and equipment. Many local organizations, hospitals, and emergency and fire rescue departments provide required semiannual certifications in BLS, ACLS, and PALS. It is important for a dental practice to recognize that skills taught semiannually may be quickly forgotten unless they are regularly practiced.[19] Therefore, a regimen of more frequent drills in shorter duration is suggested as a means to maintain skills and retain knowledge.[20] The development of a consistent in situ office training schedule that is strictly adhered to maximizes emergency preparedness of all staff members. For example, dedicating and scheduling 1 hour on the first Monday of each month with specific goals, objectives, and skills can be planned on an annual basis.

As an alternative to in situ training, many local, state, and national organizations and society-sponsored conferences offer hands-on simulation training typically open to all members of an OMS team. Another option is to contact a local hospital, college, and/or university simulation center that contracts to groups using their centers. Virtual online programs have become more common and accessible as a convenient way for dental practices to have their team members complete continuing education requirements. Insurance carriers, risk management groups, and national societies are also good resources to access for potential online continuing education opportunities. In conclusion, enhancing the emergency preparedness of an entire OMS team through simulation training sharpens skills, communication, and knowledge when responding to a medical emergency or crisis in the dental office.[21]

THE FUTURE OF SIMULATION

The future of simulation will likely involve a continued evolution from different driving forces. Health care organizations and professional societies seek to use simulation to improve learning, performance, and patient safety and assure maintenance of competency. There is no doubt that simulation will be a component in training and maintenance of skills for health care professionals. Funders of health care, liability insurers and the government seek to use simulation to reduce costs, reduce errors, and reduce claims. The future of simulation will involve 3 different models of simulation to address cost effectiveness and clinical applications. Those 3 models will be physical reality (patient mannequins), screen-based simulation, and virtual reality with either 2-D or 3-D with or without physical tools.[22] Further research is needed to clarify the best roles and cost effectiveness of simulation training in professional schools, training programs, and maintenance of competency for trained professionals.

REFERENCES

1. Tactical Combat Casualty Care – DocPlayer.net. Available at: http://www.specialoperationsmedicine. org/documents/TCCC/06%20TCCC%20Reference% 20Documents/TCCC%20Change%20Prop%201501 %20CricKey%20150603.pdf. Accessed February 12, 2017.
2. Aziz MF, Brambrink AM, Healy DW, et al. Success of intubation rescue techniques after failed direct laryngoscopy in adults: a retrospective comparative analysis from multicenter perioperative outcomes group. Anesthesiology 2016;125:656–66.
3. Lambert RC, Ban C, Rivera AU, et al. Comparison of direct laryngoscopy and videolaryngoscopy in intubating a mannequin: assessing both oral and maxillofacial surgery residents and practitioners. J Oral Maxillofac Surg 1901; 73:2015.
4. Weller JM, Merry AF, Robinson BJ, et al. The impact of trained assistance on error rates in anaesthesia: a simulation –based randomized controlled trial. Anaesthesia 2009;64:126.
5. Kluger MT, Bukofzer M, Bullock M. Anaesthetic assistants: their role in the development and resolution of anaesthetic incidents. Anaesth Intensive Care 1999;27(3):269–74.
6. Driskell JE, Salas E, Johnston J. Does stress lead to a loss of team perspective? Group Dyn 1999;3:291–302.
7. Bourne LE Jr, Yaroush RA. Stress and cognition: a cogni-tive psychological perspective. NASA technical report. 2003. Available at: http://ntrs.nasa.gov/search. jsp?R=20040034070. Accessed February 12, 2017.

8. Harrison TK, Manser T, Howard SK, et al. Use of cognitive aids in a simulated anesthetic crisis. Anesth Analg 2006;103:551–6.

9. Arriaga AF, Bader AM, Wong JM, et al. Simulation-based trial of surgical-crisis checklists. N Engl J Med 2013;368:246–53.

10. Available at: https://www.mhaus.org/PubData/PDFs/treatmentposter.pdf. Accessed October 4, 2016.

11. Wayne DB, Didwania A, Feinglass J, et al. Simulation-based education improves quality of care during cardiac arrest team responses at an academic teaching hospital: a case-controlled study. Chest 2008;133:56.

12. Office anesthesia evaluation manual. 8th edition. Rosemont (IL): AAOMS Publications; 2012. p. 41.

13. Cooper JB, Newbower RS, Long CD, et al. Preventable anesthesia mishaps: a study of human factors. Anesthesiology 1978;49:399–406.

14. Bosack RC, Lieblich S. Anesthesia complications in the dental office: anesthestic adversity, respiratory problems, vol. 32. Ames (IA): Wiley Blackwell; 2015. p. 219–30.

15. Bosack RC, Lieblich S. Anesthesia complications in the dental office: anesthestic adversity, Cardiovascular problems, vol. 33. Ames (IA): Wiley Blackwell; 2015. p. 231–49.

16. Advanced Cardiac Life Support Provider Manual. American Heart Association. Effective resuscitative team dynamics. 2011;3:17–24.

17. Internet citation: teamstepps dental module. Rockville (MD): Agency for Healthcare Research and Quality; 2015. Available at: http://www.ahrq.gov/professionals/education/curriculum-tools/teamstepps/dental/index.html. Accessed February 12, 2017.

18. Guidelines Update for CPR and ECC. American Heart Association. Adult basic life support and cardiopulmonary resuscitation quality: systems of care: 2015; Part 4 p. S405. Available at: http://eccguidelines.heart.org/wp-content/uploads/2015/10/2015-AHA-Guidelines-Highlights-English.pdf. Accessed January 12, 2017.

19. Kurek MM, Devih JH, Cohen M. Cardiac in the OR: how are our ACLS skills? Can J Anaesth 1998;45:130–2.

20. Levy JH, The American Society of Anesthesiologists, Inc. Lippincott Williams & Wilkins. This is not a test:. misconceptions surrounding the maintenance of certification in anesthesiology simulation course. Anesthesiology 2014;121:655–9.

21. Lufty-Clayton L, Staying sharp with simulation: emergency physicians monthly. 2012.

22. Gaba DM. The future vision of simulation in health care. Qual Saf Health Care 2004;13(Suppl 1):i2–10.

Fire Safety for the Oral and Maxillofacial Surgeon and Surgical Staff

LisaMarie Di Pasquale, DDS, MD[a],
Elie M. Ferneini, DMD, MD, MHS, MBA[a,b,c],*

KEYWORDS

- Fire safety • Fire prevention • Fire management • Patient safety • Surgical fires

KEY POINTS

- Fire in the operating room is a life-threatening emergency that demands quick and efficient intervention.
- Because the circumstances surrounding fires are generally well-understood, virtually every operating room fire is preventable.
- Before every operating room case, thorough preprocedure "time outs" should address each team members' awareness of specific fire risks and agreement regarding fire concerns and emergency actions.
- Fire prevention largely centers on recognition by all surgical team members of the 3 constituent parts of the fire triad necessary for fire formation.
- Regular fire drills should guide in developing policies and procedures to prevent surgical fires; delivering optimal patient care in emergent situations requires surgical team training, practicing emergency roles and specific actions.

INTRODUCTION

Fires in the operating room are unanticipated, devastating events that can lead to significant morbidity, even mortality, for the patient and medical personnel. The actual incidence of fires is difficult to quantify. Currently, in the United States there is no federal requirement for reporting a surgical fire and no centralized archive exists that classifies the total number of fires.[1–5] Estimates state as few as 100 and as many as 650 operating room fires occur annually in the United States.[3,6] Results from studies at the ECRI Institute and the US Food and Drug Administration estimate that operating room fires cause approximately 20 serious patient injuries to occur annually, with 1 to 2 deaths per year.[3,7,8]

Despite scrupulous attention to patient safety, the incidence of operating room fires does not seem to be decreasing.[7] In 2008, the Joint Commission on Accreditation of Healthcare Organizations (JCAHO) made reducing the incidence of surgical fires a targeted initiative. Noting the unique environment of the operating room and the extreme morbidity often caused by surgical fires, JCAHO declared the need for "response and prevention strategies to be specific to the setting."[5]

As oral and maxillofacial surgeons, the topic of fire safety demands attention and preparedness. Approximately 78% of all fires occur during facial, neck, and tonsil surgery.[9] In addition, understanding fire safety and prevention measures, as well as protocol and management of an actual fire, are

a Division of Oral and Maxillofacial Surgery, Department of Craniofacial Sciences, University of Connecticut, 263 Farmington Avenue, Farmington, CT 06030, USA; b Private Practice, Greater Waterbury OMS, 435 Highland Avenue, Suite 100, Cheshire, CT 06410, USA; c Beau Visage Med Spa, 435 Highland Avenue, Suite 100, Cheshire, CT 06410, USA
* Corresponding author. Beau Visage Med Spa, 435 Highland Avenue, Suite 100, Cheshire, CT 06410, USA.
E-mail address: eferneini@yahoo.com

Oral Maxillofacial Surg Clin N Am 29 (2017) 179–187
http://dx.doi.org/10.1016/j.coms.2016.12.004
1042-3699/17/© 2016 Elsevier Inc. All rights reserved.

necessary for all operating room staff.[7] The most prevailing matter with surgical fires is that they are nearly always preventable.[3] All members of the surgical team must understand the root cause and the constituent parts in the outbreak of a fire to prevent the catastrophe. With proper fire safety and prevention training for all operating room personnel and with the use of proper surgical technique, fires simply should not occur.[7]

CAUSES OF FIRE

Fires can occur in any setting, provided these 3 elements are in close proximity under the right conditions: (1) heat or an ignition source, (2) fuel, and (3) an oxidizer.[10,11] Patients are at greatest risk of fire injury when all 3 elements of the fire triad are in close vicinity.[12,13] Unfortunately, the oxygen-rich atmosphere, flammable materials, and ignition sources are abundant in the operating room and routinely a part of the sterile field.[3,12] Specific to oral and maxillofacial surgery, objects with potential for ignition are often in close proximity to multiple fuel sources in a confined environment with high levels of circulating oxidizing agents.[6] The fire triad is interdependent; thus, eliminating any 1 element removes the potential of a fire outbreak altogether.[7] Fire safety is everyone's responsibility and each component can be controlled to a certain degree by either the surgeon, the anesthesia provider, and/or nursing team members.[12]

IGNITION SOURCES

The most common ignition source cited in operating room fires is the electrosurgical unit, which is used in approximately 85% of surgeries; supplemental oxygen was also present in most cases.[5,14] Lasers are another common ignition source, and even the extreme heat generated by the high-intensity (fiber-optic) light cords can serve as an ignition source.[10] The electric surgical unit produces heat by concentrating electrical current at the tip of the electrode, which can reach several hundred degrees. If this occurs in an oxygen-rich environment or if a fuel source is present, a fire may result.[1,5] Orofacial surgery creates just such an environment, and if these instruments are used, they may potentially ignite endotracheal tubes, possibly starting a fire in the airway itself.[3] Other standard operating room equipment, such as light cables and boxes, drills, saws, burs, argon beam coagulators, and defibrillators may all serve as potential ignition sources.[3]

FUEL SOURCES

The modern-day operating room is full of available fuel sources (**Box 1**). The most obvious are linens, prepping agents, dressings, and even personal protective equipment, which can easily burn.[7] Only the water-based preparation solutions, such as betadine, contain no alcohol and can be considered nonflammable.[5] However, most of the current preparation solutions contain some alcohol, and flammability is directly related to their alcohol concentration.[5,7] Surgeons should allow alcohol-based skin preparation solutions sufficient time to dry before draping the patient.[7] Although 2 to 3 minutes is recommended often, a total of 5 minutes should be allowed to pass to permit the alcohol content to evaporate.[5] In addition, ointments, tinctures, and degreasers such as mastisol or benzoin can serve as another potentially combustible fuel source because they are made of high concentrations of alcohol.[5]

The patient's body itself can provide numerous fuel sources. Gastrointestinal gases (methane, hydrogen), desiccated tissue, and hair are a few elements that can support fire. In the past, combustible anesthetic gases were used widely and thus often functioned as a fuel supply.[7]

Surgical equipment burns readily, including tourniquet cuffs, tubing, wound drains, drapes, and packing materials. Even drapes that are labeled as 'nonflammable' can be a fuel source in an environment that promotes fire.[5] One study that evaluated surgical drapes found the higher the oxygen concentration in the room, the faster the nonflammable drapes would ignite and burn. Interestingly, if the oxygen level was high enough, flammable and nonflammable drapes had nearly identical combustion times.[15]

Despite the obvious devastation of a surgical fire burn, another factor in injury is the toxic chemicals produced by the combustion of materials.[7] Potentially hazardous fumes such as carbon monoxide, ammonia, and cyanide may result from the ignition of medical equipment. These toxic byproducts pose an additional harm to patients and staff.

OXIDIZER

Oxidizers are substances that lower the temperature at which a fuel will ignite, thus increasing the chance of a fire.[10] The primary oxidizer in the operating room is oxygen itself.[3] Nitrous oxide should not be disregarded as an oxidizer agent. When heated, nitrous oxide decomposes into its constituent elements, thereby increasing the ambient oxygen.[7,10] Nitrous oxide can also support combustion by exothermal dissociation, thereby releasing heat and oxygen. In fact, fires involving oxygen and/or nitrous oxide mixtures can be as severe as those involving 100% oxygen. In the operating room, the ignition source is generally

> **Box 1**
> **Fuel sources in the operating room**
>
> - Ointments and solutions
> - Patient sources
> - Materials
> - Equipment
> - "Prep" solutions (alcohol, chlorhexidine, Duraprep)
> - Tinctures (benzoin, mastisol, merthiolate)
> - Degreasers (acetone, ether)
> - Petrolatum and petrolatum-based dressings/ointments
> - Visible hair
> - Lanugo (invisible hair)
> - Gastrointestinal gases (methane, hydrogen)
> - Desiccated tissue
> - Drapes (on the patient or on equipment, paper, plastic, cloth)
> - Dressings (gauze, Xeroform, sponges, tape, ace bandages)
> - Gowns, caps, masks, shoe covers, gloves
> - Anesthesia (endotracheal tubes, breathing circuits, masks, suction catheters, oral/nasal airways, intravenous tubing, laryngeal mask airways, scavenger tubes, coverings of cables/wires)
> - Surgical (fiberoptic cable/wire coverings, pneumatic tourniquet cuffs/tubing, wound drains/collections systems, steri-drapes, disposable packing materials).[3]
>
> *Adapted from* Rinder CS. Fire safety in the operating room. Curr Opin Anaesthesiol 2008;21(6):791; with permission.

controlled by the surgeon and the oxygen source typically controlled by the anesthetist.[1] As such, the anesthesiologist must choose an anesthetic technique based on the surgical procedure that is being done and must balance risk of hypoxia, by lowering the fraction of inspired oxygen (Fio_2), with that of fire safety.[6] Because oxygen and nitrous oxide are both oxidizers that have no color or odor, it is essential to communicate with the surgeon frequently during the procedure regarding the use of these combustible gases.[7] Specifically with the airway, if the endotracheal tube filled with oxygen or nitrous oxide is ignited, flames are directed down the tube directly into the trachea. Additionally, endotracheal tubes with cuffs should be used because the cuff helps to create a seal and minimizes oxygen leaks.[7,16,17]

One study found that oxygen flow rates and Fio_2 are inversely related to the amount of time it takes to ignite a fire in an oropharyngeal surgical model. Although a fire was easily started when using 100% Fio_2, a longer exposure to an ignition source was required for ignition as the amount of Fio_2 decreased. In fact, an Fio_2 of less than 50% in the oropharyngeal surgical models could not support an ignition or actual flames.[6] Thus, for decreased risk of fire, the Fio_2 should be less than 30% whenever possible during open oxygen delivery, particularly if electrocautery or a laser is being used.[5,7,12]

Of note are monitored anesthesia care cases with the use of nasal cannula oxygen. In most monitored anesthesia care cases of a fire, supplemental oxygen was used. Ninety-five percent of cases involved the head or neck, whereas alcohol-containing preparation solutions and/or drapes were the most common fuel sources.[5] Owing to regulated mechanisms for air exchange in the operating room, the delivery of 100% oxygen through the cannula at flow rates of 1 to 6 L/min do not typically produce enough of an oxidizing agent to cause a significant fire hazard.[5] The flow rate of the supplemental oxygen, such as a nasal cannula, should be set to the lowest possible setting to reduce unnecessary excess oxygen while still maintaining safe blood oxygenation saturation levels.[7,12] If electrocautery or laser is being used, oxygen administration should be replaced with medical grade air.

Furthermore, patient draping may be a significant factor in oxygen dispersal, because draping around the patient's head, particularly in head and neck surgery may form an "occlusive tent."[5] If the patient is draped before preparation solutions have dried, the drapes may tent the vapors in the surgical field. At this point, any ignition source may easily lead to a fire.[7,18]

MANAGEMENT OF A FIRE

It is the responsibility of all health care personnel to protect patients and staff, and to avoid the destruction of a surgical fire. Everyone plays a vital role in fire safety, prevention, and control.[12] Often, the RACE method is used to guide actions when a fire occurs. This fire protection mnemonic stands for

- Rescue,
- Alarm,
- Confine/contain, and
- Extinguish.[12]

Rescue

In the event of a fire, rescue simply means to move patients out of harm's way. The first step in the "rescue" algorithm is to stop all airway gases immediately and ensure safety for the patient and all members of the team.

Alarm or Alert

The person who notices the fire should call out and alert others to the situation. The anesthetist, the operating room staff, and the surgeon work together once the fire is identified. The surgeon determines the point at which it is safe to stop the procedure and ensure hemostasis, and the rest of the team establishes how and where to move the patient.

Confine or Contain

The initial safety actions should be to ensure patient safety. After the movement of patients in the immediate danger of the fire, personnel should work to contain the fire to prevent smoke and fire from entering other operating rooms.

Extinguish

Extinguishing the fire is important in any fire management. However, in the event of an airway fire, smothering the flames serves to save the patient as well as manage the fire. To extinguish a fire, 3 types of portable extinguishers are available: ABC, carbon dioxide, and water mist.

ABC extinguishers are used for ordinary combustible materials, flammable liquids, and electrical fires (**Box 2**). Carbon dioxide extinguishers are used for flammable liquids and electrical fires. Water-mist extinguishers, which contain deionized water, are used for ordinary

---

> **Box 2**
> **National Fire Protection Association standards for classification of the different types of fire extinguishers**
>
> - Class A: for use on wood, paper, cloth, and most plastics (eg, combustible materials);
> - Class B: for use on flammable liquids or grease; and
> - Class C: for use on energized electrical equipment.[3]

---

combustibles and energized electrical fires. All fire extinguishers used in the operating room are of the ABC variety, meaning that they are effective in fighting all types of fires (ordinary combustibles, flammable liquids, and electrical fires). When the patient is the fuel source, such as in an airway fire, a CO_2 extinguisher should be used because it lacks ammonium phosphate, the dry chemical fire retardant that can be corrosive to the patient's tissues. Proper use involves the PASS (pull pin, aim, squeeze, and sweep) technique. The PASS method serves as a useful reminder for using a fire extinguisher appropriately (**Fig. 1**).[12]

ROLES

All operating room personnel (surgeons, anesthetists, surgical technicians, nurses, students) should be trained in fire safety procedures. Responsibility for each contributing factor to the fire triad lies with each member of the surgical team. The anesthesiologist is generally in charge of supplying and monitoring the oxidizing agents, the surgeon is largely responsible for ignition sources in the surgical field, and nurses usually look after the materials in the operating room. Proper training should be given to all members of the surgical team that includes an explanation and understanding of the designated roles in the event of a fire. It is essential that operating room staff become familiar with the different classes of fire extinguishers and trained on how to use them.[7] In addition to learning equipment, role responsibilities, and emergency preparedness, fire drills should be conducted to ensure proficiency of the staff with the safety plan.[7,19]

PREPARATION

The best method of fighting a fire is to avoid having one in the first place. Great emphasis should be placed on prevention.[1] Education and training

Pull the safety pin from the handle.

Aim the extinguisher at the base of the fire, not at the flames.

Squeeze the handles slowly together to discharge the extinguishing agent.

Sweep side-to-side in a sweeping motion until expended, keeping a safe distance from the fire.

Fig. 1. The PASS (pull pin, aim, squeeze, and sweep) method. PASS refers to a fire-prevention mnemonic for recalling the steps in correct fire extinguisher use. (*From* Seifert PC, Peterson E, Graham K. Crisis management of fire in the OR. AORN J 2015;101(2):258; with permission.)

in fire risk reduction strategies for perioperative nurses, surgical technicians, anesthetists, and surgeons is essential to promoting and maintaining a fire safe environment (**Box 3**). To promote fire prevention and plan an effective response, it is important to hold fire safety drills and exercises on how to manage the fire safely and efficiently (**Box 4**).[12] In fact, an operating room fire safety drill is a formal and periodic rehearsal of the operating room team's planned response to a fire.

Initial safety evaluations should aim to test the availability and functional status of the operating room fire safety equipment. Surgical team personnel know the location of fire extinguishers, and fire alarms, gas valves, airway protection equipment, and flashlights should be visibly marked and easily accessible.[20]

One of the most essential, yet often overlooked factors in fire prevention, is intraoperative communication among members of the surgical team.[7] As mentioned, oropharyngeal and facial surgery, in particular, places all components of the fire triad in close proximity and undoubtedly increases the likelihood of combustion. For this reason, a preoperative discussion among the surgical team, often part of the "time out," should be completed to classify the fire risk level of the planned procedure.[7] Additionally, effective communication between the surgeon and anesthesia provider is critical, especially when fire is a risk. The surgeon should inform the anesthesia provider when electrocautery is being used; this way, the anesthesia provider can adjust the oxygen. Before the start of the surgery, a time out procedure would have ideally defined the predetermined fire safety responsibilities for each member of the surgical team. The fire risk scale is from 0 (very low risk) to 3 (high risk), with 1 point given for each of the following: surgical site above the xiphoid, open oxygen source, and use of ignition source. In the case of a high fire risk, denoted with a score

of 3, the team should create a plan to minimize fire risk by taking the proper precautions.[21]

MANAGEMENT

Although smoke, heat, and flames usually indicate the presence of a fire, occasionally it presents with unfamiliar sounds and odors.[7] Surgical team

---

Box 3
Operating room staff actions to prevent fires

Training programs should include details on the role-specific actions that are to be taken by the operating room staff to prevent fires. Examples include:

- Keep the electrocautery tip in a holster when it is not being used.
- Turn off all high-intensity light sources when not in use.
- Using cuffed endotracheal tubes, and appropriate use of oxygen gas.
- Beware of patient draping so as to not create occlusive "tent" to trap in oxidizing agents.
- Attempt to use water-soluble preparation solutions and ointments.
- Consider flame resistant surgical drapes.
- Know the location of the fire extinguishers, alarms, and gas valves.
- Obtain proficiency with fire extinguishers and equipment.
- Know the location of all fire alarm and fire exits.[1]

Every fire safety exercise should be considered a beneficial learning experience for all staff members. Surgical team preparedness will help to strengthen efficient safety response in the event of a fire.[3]
Data from Association of periOperative Registered Nurses. AORN guidance statement: fire prevention in the operating room. AORN J 2005;81(5):1067–75.

Box 4
Key points in planning a fire drill

- Choosing a date and time
- Developing a well-thought-out scenario(s)
- Completing a fire drill record participants and pertinent details
- Identifying observers and their locations
- Designating surgical team members who will participate in the event and briefing them on the scenario
- Reviewing fire safety/drill policy and procedures and their roles with staff members
- Discussing the drill in a debriefing session, identifying areas for improvement and areas of strength
- Evaluating the effectiveness of the staff-members and equipment used

---

members should heed these unusual occurrences and not dismiss the clues that something is burning. Surgery should be paused and it should be established if a fire exists, or if there is a potential fire threat to safety.[7]

The roles of the surgical team may be assigned as follows. Within the operating room, the circulating nurse should ensure patient safety by remaining with the patient while activating the fire alarm system and alerting all necessary personnel. The nurse will be able to provide the scrub technician and anesthetist with needed supplies to extinguish the flames. Additionally, if anything is burning near the patient, the nurse can help remove it and extinguish the flaming material with water. Because optimum patient safety may require moving the patient from the operating room, the nurse should obtain a transport stretcher and prepare the patient for transporting out of the operating room.

Another nurse, often in the perioperative area, should notify the hospital emergency response team of a fire and its location. Additional pertinent details are important to communicate, such as other operating rooms at risk and condition of at-risk patients who may also require immediate evacuation.

The surgical scrub technician has the primary responsibility of removing flammable materials from around the patient. The surgeon should be assisted in dressing the surgical wound, if applicable, and help to prepare and transport the patient from the operating room.

Once the fire has been identified, the surgery should be stopped and hemostasis achieved. The surgeon will achieve this by attending to the wounds and dressing them appropriately. Furthermore, the fire safety role of the surgeon includes removing flammable materials from around the patient and helping to extinguish the fire. If the patient is being prepared for evacuation, it is up to the surgeon to decide if the patient is in immediate

danger from a procedural standpoint and to help move the patient if necessary.

The anesthetist should immediately shut off the oxidizing agents, such as oxygen and nitrous oxide, in the event of a fire. If the fire is in the patient's airway, the patient will be quickly extubated and the anesthetist is to maintain breathing for the patient with a valve mask respirator. The circulating nurse may be instructed to turn off the gas shutoff valves. The patient should be reintubated once the fire is extinguished. In the event of patient evacuation, the anesthetist will help to disconnect any lines and equipment from the patient. Also, because the patient may be under general anesthesia, the anesthetist must gather necessary medications to continue anesthesia and support the patient during transport.

If necessary, patients should be evacuated quickly from the operating room to a safe area nearby. Surgical team members should know the location of all fire exits and ensure that these exits are clear for evacuation.[3] All members of the surgical team should be accounted for by a head count. After evacuation of the room, everything should be left in place so the fire department can conduct their investigation of the cause of the fire.[3,5] **Fig. 2** reviews a fire management algorithm.[22]

TYPES OF FIRES

Categorically, operating room fires may be divided into fires occurring on the patient, including airway fires, and fires away from the patient that occur within the operating room. Regardless of the type of fire, the first priority is extinguishing the flames and removing the burning material from near or on the patient.[10]

If the fire is not located on the patient, if possible the flaming material should be removed and extinguished outside of the operating room. However, if the flammable object is unable to be removed from

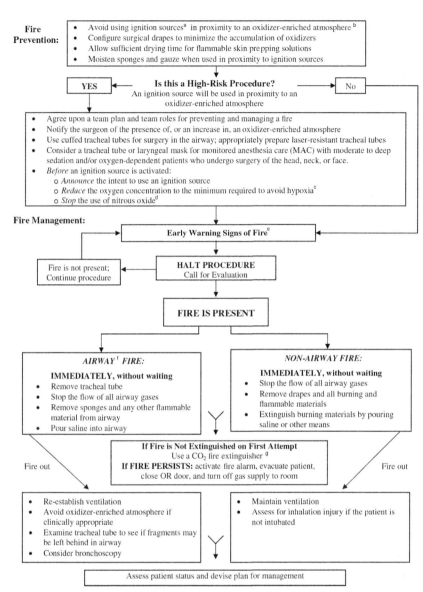

Fig. 2. Operating room (OR) fires algorithm. [a] Ignition sources include but are not limited to electrosurgery or electrocautery units and lasers. [b] An oxidizer-enriched atmosphere occurs when there is any increase in oxygen concentration above room air level, and/or the presence of any concentration of nitrous oxide. [c] After minimizing delivered oxygen, wait a period of time (eg, 1–3 min) before using an ignition source. For oxygen dependent patients, *reduce* supplemental oxygen delivery to the minimum required to avoid hypoxia. Monitor oxygenation with pulse oximetry, and if feasible, inspired, exhaled, and/or delivered oxygen concentration. [d] After stopping the delivery of nitrous oxide, wait a period of time (eg, 1–3 min) before using an ignition source. [e] Unexpected flash, flame, smoke or heat, unusual sounds (eg, a "pop," snap or "foomp") or odors, unexpected movement of drapes, discoloration of drapes or breathing circuit, unexpected patient movement or complaint. [f] In this algorithm, airway fire refers to a fire in the airway or breathing circuit. [g] A CO_2 fire extinguisher may be used on the patient if necessary. (*From* Apfelbaum JL, Caplan RA, Barker SJ, et al. Practice advisory for the prevention and management of operating room fires. An updated report by the American Society of Anesthesiologists task force on operating room fires. Anesthesiology 2013;118(2):276; with permission.)

the operating room, or unable to be controlled with saline or water alone, a fire extinguisher should be used to put out the fire.[10]

The circulating nurse, or whoever is designated, should activate the fire alarm and alert the emergency services of the hospital.[7]

If the burning object is located on or inside the patient, smoldering material should be removed and the flames should be extinguished with water or sterile saline. All gases and oxidizing agents such as oxygen and nitrous oxide should be discontinued immediately and any flaming material

Box 5
Equipment and supplies that should be immediately available if fires are a risk

- Several containers of sterile saline
- A carbon dioxide fire extinguisher
- Replacement tracheal tubes, guides, face masks
- Rigid laryngoscope blades; this may include a rigid fiberoptic laryngoscope
- Replacement airway breathing circuits and lines
- Replacement drapes, sponges

submerged in water.[7] If it is an airway fire, all gases are discontinued at the first sign of flames. The anesthetist will then make the decision to extubate the patient and ventilate the patient with air until the flames are controlled. As with any fire, burning items are removed from the patient and extinguished. The patient should be reintubated with judicious use of oxygen as soon as safely possible.[10,23]

Fire alarms, monitored smoke detectors, and heat sensors are located throughout the hospital. A circulating nurse or available surgical team member must activate the alarms via the pull stations, which are often located near exits and stairwells. The response team includes but is not limited to security and facility management personnel. On their arrival, they determine what additional resources are required and whether evacuation of the area is necessary.[10]

Shutoff valves are used to stop the flow of gases into the operating rooms. The shutoff valves should be accessed in the hallways and pulled into the off position.[10] Surgical team members must be familiar with the location of gas shutoff valve location and turn them off if designated by their predetermined fire safety role.[3]

Once the flames are extinguished, if it is possible to control the immediate danger, attention should be directed to the potential damage caused by the smoke. If the fire is unable to be contained expediently, then evacuation efforts should be made for the patient and surgical team. Immediate notification of the fire department should occur.[10] After the fire, the room should be left intact so that the fire department can complete a thorough evaluation into the cause of the fire (**Box 5**).[7,22]

SUMMARY

Fire in the operating room is a life-threatening emergency that demands quick and efficient intervention.[12] Because the circumstances surrounding

fires are generally well-understood, virtually every operating room fire is preventable.[10] Before every operating room case, thorough preprocedure "time outs" should address each surgical team members' awareness of the specific fire risks and agreement regarding fire-concerns and emergency actions.[10] Fire prevention largely centers on recognition by all surgical team members of the 3 constituent parts of the fire triad necessary for fire formation.[5] Regular fire drills should guide in developing policies and procedures that will prevent surgical fires.[3] Delivering optimal patient care in emergent situations requires surgical team training, practicing emergency roles, and specific actions that are essential to a coordinated and smooth emergency response.[12]

Unfortunately, airway fires remain a significant risk for patients undergoing orofacial surgery.[6] Maxillofacial procedures in particular present the risk of fire because of the use of supplemental oxygen, surgical instrumentation, and ignition sources, while in the presence of flammable materials.[6]

Operating room fires are uncommon, but have the potential for catastrophic outcomes.[5] Anesthesiologists are responsible for the management of oxidizing agents being used, such as supplemental oxygen, particularly in operations on the head and neck. Surgeons and operating room nurses need to be conscious of preparation solutions and ointments they use. Also, exercising fire safe practices with electrosurgical units and lasers, using good communication with the anesthetist regarding their use around oxygen sources and flammable agents are essential. Surgical team members must display proficient knowledge of the location of fire extinguishers, fire alarms, and gas shutoff valves.[7] With the preventable nature of surgical fires, it is vital that the surgical team understands the essentials of fire safety, prevention, and management to see a decrease in the frequency of fires.[7] Surgical fires have the potential for high morbidity and mortality and the goal for the surgical team is to minimize this risk.

REFERENCES

1. Norris J. Fire safety in the operating room. AANA J 1994;62(4):342–5. Available at: https://www.aana.com/newsandjournal/Documents/fire_safety_0894_p342.pdf. Accessed January 12, 2016.
2. Meneghetti S, Morgan M, Fritz J, et al. Operating room fires: optimizing safety. Plast Reconstr Surg 2007;120(6):1701–8.
3. Association of periOperative Registered Nurses. AORN guidance statement: fire prevention in the operating room. AORN J 2005;81(5):1067–75.

4. Corvetto M, Hobbs G, Taekman J. Fire in the operating room. Simulation Healthc 2011;6(6):356–9.

5. Rinder CS. Fire safety in the operating room. Curr Opin Anaesthesiology 2008;21(6):790–5.

6. Soham R, Smith LP. What does it take to start an oropharyngeal fire? Oxygen requirements to start fires in the operating room. Int J Pediatr Otorhinolaryngol 2011;75(2):227–30.

7. Kaye A, Kolinsky D, Urman R. Management of a fire in the operating room. J Anesth 2014;28(2):279–87. Available at: http://link.springer.com/article/10.1007/s00540-013-1705-6. Accessed January 12, 2016.

8. ECRI. New clinical guidance for surgical fire prevention. Health Devices 2009;38(10):314–32.

9. Daane SP, Toth BA. Fire in the operating room: principles and prevention. Plast Reconstr Surg 2005;115(5):73e–5e.

10. Hart SR, Yajnik A, Ashford J, et al. Operating room fire safety. The Ochsner J 2011;11(1):37–42.

11. Engel S, Patel NK, Morrison CM, et al. Operating room fires. Plast Reconstr Surg 2012;130(3):681–9.

12. Seifert PC, Peterson E, Graham K. Crisis management of fire in the OR. AORN J 2015;101(2):250–63.

13. ECRI Institute. Devastation of patient fires. Health Devices 1992;21:3–39.

14. Preventing surgical fires. Sentinel Event Alert 29 (June 24, 2003). Available at: http://www.jointcommission.org/sentinel_event_alert_issue_29_preventing_surgical_fires/. Accessed January 12, 2016.

15. Golderberg J. Brief laboratory report: surgical drape flammability. AANA J 2006;75(4):352–4.

16. Hermens JH, Bennett MJ, Hirshman CA. Anesthesia for laser surgery. Anesth Analg 1983;62(2):218–29.

17. Riefkohl R, Kosanin RM. A practical method for oxygen administration during cosmetic facial surgery. Ann Plast Surg 1986;16(6):535–7.

18. Prasad R, Quezado Z, Andre AS, et al. Fires in the operating room and intensive care unit: awareness is the key to prevention. Anesth Analg 2006;102(1):172–4.

19. Greco RJ, Gonzalez R, Johnson P, et al. Potential dangers of oxygen supplementation during facial surgery. Plast Reconstr Surg 1995;95(6):978–84.

20. Barash PG, Cullen BF, Stoelting RK, et al. Chapter 8: fire safety. Clinical anesthesia. 6th edition. Philadelphia: Lippincott Williams & Wilkins; 2009.

21. Steelman VM, Hottel RA. Where there's smoke, there's…. AORN J 2009;89(5):825–7.

22. Apfelbaum JL, Caplan RA, Barker SJ, et al. Practice advisory for the prevention and management of operating room fires. An updated report by the American Society of Anesthesiologists task force on operating room fires. Anesthesiology 2013;118(2):271–90.

23. Mathias JM. Scoring fire risk for surgical patients. OR Manag 2006;22(1):19.

Outpatient Anesthetic Safety Considerations for Obstructive Sleep Apnea

Kevin J. Butterfield, MD, DDS*

KEYWORDS

- Obstructive sleep apnea • Outpatient anesthesia • STOP-BANG questionnaire
- Diagnosing obstructive sleep apnea • Patient safety

KEY POINTS

- Most patients with obstructive sleep apnea (OSA) are not diagnosed preoperatively.
- The STOP-BANG questionnaire may identify patients at risk of OSA, especially those with severe OSA.
- Patients with mild to moderate OSA, with optimized comorbidities, can usually safely undergo outpatient surgery.
- Patients with severe OSA, who are not optimized medically, should avoid outpatient surgery.

The perioperative management of patients with OSA is challenging, rewarding and is appropriate to be included in an issue dedicated to patient safety. OSA is a chronic condition in which intermittent and recurrent episodes of partial or complete obstruction of the upper airway occur during sleep. These episodes disrupt sleep architecture, causing fragmented sleep and daytime sleepiness, and result in recurrent oxyhemoglobin desaturations. Left untreated, these episodes may result in significant morbidity and mortality.[1–8] Up to 34% of men and 17% of women meet the polysomnographic criteria to diagnose OSA.[9] An obstructive apnea is defined as the absence of airflow for at least 10 seconds despite ventilatory efforts, whereas an obstructive hypopnea is defined as a 30% (or greater) reduction in airflow lasting for 10 seconds or longer and an associated 4% (or greater) oxyhemoglobin desaturation level or if it results in arousal or fragmentation of sleep. OSA is defined as an apnea-hypopnea index (AHI) greater than or equal to 5 with associated symptoms, such as daytime sleepiness, fatigue, or impaired cognition, or an AHI greater than or equal to 15 without associated symptoms. OSA severity is categorized as follows: 5 to 14 = mild, 15 to 29 = moderate, and greater than 30 = severe.

OSA is associated with significant comorbidities, as described in **Table 1**.[5–7,10] Moderate to severe OSA is associated with increases in hypertension, strokes, atrial fibrillation, sudden cardiac death, and reduced left ventricular function in heart failure. It is associated with hyperglycemia in diabetic patients, impaired cognitive function, and increased risk for automobile accidents,[1] all-cause mortality, and cancer.[11]

Recently, numerous studies[7,15,21] have shown that OSA patients have an increased risk of having perioperative complications, including pneumonia, hypoxemia, difficult intubation, pulmonary embolism, myocardial infarction, atelectasis, cardiac arrhythmias, and unanticipated admission to an intensive care unit. Most patients with OSA

Division of Dentistry/Oral and Maxillofacial Surgery, Department of Otolaryngology, Ottawa Hospital, University of Ottawa School of Medicine, Ottawa, Ontario, Canada
* 499 Terry Fox Drive, Unit 15, Kanata, Ontario K2T-1H7, Canada.
E-mail address: kbutterfield@toh.ca

Oral Maxillofacial Surg Clin N Am 29 (2017) 189–196
http://dx.doi.org/10.1016/j.coms.2016.12.007

Table 1
Coexisting diseases/symptoms associated with obstructive sleep apnea

Cardiovascular	% of Patients with Obstructive Sleep Apnea	Endocrine/Other	% of Patients with Obstructive Sleep Apnea
Drug-resistant HTN[12]	83	Glucose intolerance/ diabetes[13]	48
Arrhythmias[14]	49	Obesity[15]	77
Coronary artery disease[16]	30	Gastroesophageal reflux disease[17]	46
Myocardial infarction[18]	6	Cancer[18]	3
Congestive heart failure[19]	36	—	—
COPD[18]	24	—	—
Peripheral vascular disease[18]	4	—	—
Pulmonary hypertension[18]	3	—	—
Pacemaker[20]	59	—	—

Data from Refs.[12,14,16,18–20]

are undiagnosed at the time of admission. Therefore, it is important to identify these patients preoperatively so that appropriate perioperative management protocols can be initiated.

PREOPERATIVE MANAGEMENT
Does the Patient Have Obstructive Sleep Apnea?

OSA is more prevalent in surgical patients than in the general population,[22] and the incidence of undiagnosed OSA in surgical patients has been reported as between 21% and 28%.[23,24] Unfortunately, 60% of anesthesia providers and 92% of surgeons fail to identify patients with preexisting or undiagnosed moderate to severe OSA.[2,25–29]

Three questionnaires (Berlin, American Society of Anesthesiologists [ASA], and STOP-BANG) have been validated for use in the surgical population. Of these, the STOP-BANG questionnaire was found to have the highest methodological validity.[23] It is a simple, self-administered, concise questionnaire that consists of 8 yes/no questions.[23]

The mnemonic STOP includes the following:

1. S: Do you snore loudly, loud enough to be heard through a closed door?
2. T: Do you feel tired or fatigued during the daytime almost every day?
3. O: Has anyone observed that you stop breathing during sleep?
4. P: Do you have a history of high blood pressure with or without treatment?

If a patient answers yes to more than 2 questions, the sensitivity of having an AHI greater than 5 is 66% and the sensitivity of having an AHI greater than 15 is 74%.

The mnemonic Bang is also useful, as follows:

- B: Body mass index (BMI) greater than 35
- A: Age older than 50 years
- N: Neck circumference greater than 43 cm (17 in)
- G: Gender, male

Patients are considered at high risk of OSA syndrome if they answer yes to 3 or more items (**Table 2**).

As a result, if a patient is deemed low risk for OSA using the STOP-BANG questionnaire, a clinician can be confident that the patient does not have moderate to severe OSA.

Overnight Versus Home Polysomnogram

Overnight polysomnography (PSG) is considered the gold standard for diagnosing OSA.[30,31] It is time consuming, however, and there are often long waiting periods at many centers. Consequently, unattended portable monitoring (PM) has been increasingly used for the diagnosis of OSA.[31] Unattended sleep studies have a higher failure rate (10%–20%) secondary to technical issues[32]; a negative PM study does not definitively rule out OSA[33]; and studies in broad populations comparing its effectiveness to PSG are lacking.[34] Most PM studies include a minimum of 4 parameters, including oxygen saturation, measurement of heart rate or an ECG, and at least 2 channels assessing respiration (eg, respiratory movement and airflow).[34] Recognizing the significant

Table 2
STOP-BANG questionnaire sensitivity and negative predictive value for diagnosing obstructive sleep apnea

Apnea-Hypopnea Index	Sensitivity (%)	Negative Predictive Value (%)
>5	83.6	60.8
>15	92.9	90.2
>30	100	100

Sensitivity = test's ability to correctly detect patients who do have the condition.
   Negative predictive value = probability that patients with a negative screening test truly do not have the disease.
   Data from Chung F, Yegneswaran B, Liao P, et al. STOP questionnaire: a tool to screen patients for obstructive sleep apnea. Anesthesiology 2008;108(5):812–21.

limitations to the use of PM, a task force[31] published clinical guidelines for the use of unattended PMs in the diagnosis of OSA in adult patients. The task force recommends, among other things, that PM may be used as an alternative to PSG for the diagnosis of OSA in patients with a high pretest probability of moderate to severe OSA. It is inappropriate, however, for the diagnosis of OSA in patients with significant comorbid medical conditions, because they may have a negative impact on PM's clinical accuracy. A recent review article[34] provides an excellent summary on current PM options available and an extensive discussion of its limitations. In general, PSG remains the gold standard, and if possible, should be used to diagnose and determine the severity of OSA prior to providing anesthesia.

Clinical Assessment

The general physical examination is frequently normal in patients with OSA. Clinicians should always perform an evaluation of the upper airway in all patients, particularly in nonobese adults with symptoms consistent with OSA.

Clinical findings that increase the risk of a patient presenting with OSA include[35]

- Obesity – BMI greater than 30 kg/m^2
- Increased neck circumference (>43 cm [17 in], male; 37 cm [15 in], female)
- Increased Mallampati score
- Encroachment of the lateral airway walls (independent predictor of OSA)[36]
- Increased overjet
- High-arched hard palate
- Tonsillar enlargement
- Mandibular retrognathism

Where to Provide Care?

Unfortunately, there is a paucity of literature to guide clinicians regarding which patients can be safely managed on an outpatient basis as opposed to an inpatient basis or how long patients should be monitored in a surgical facility.[22] Outpatient oral and maxillofacial surgery typically involves a nonintubated patient with an unprotected airway. As such, early and aggressive management of potential airway compromise is mandatory to prevent serious and potentially fatal complications. When deciding on treating OSA patients in a private office setting versus an ambulatory surgery center/hospital, the decision is best made preoperatively at a separate consultation appointment. It should be based on several considerations, including OSA severity; type of planned anesthetic; extent of the surgical procedure; need for postoperative narcotics; and the skill, experience, and resources available for aggressive airway management for the anesthetic team. There is an absence of rigid guidelines regarding the preferred location for providing care to OSA patients. The decision is ultimately left up to the treating clinician, taking into consideration all pertinent clinical factors to provide the most ideal outcome possible.

Use of Preoperative Continuous Positive Airway Pressure

Preoperative continuous positive airway pressure (CPAP) use has been shown to result in a lower frequency of postoperative complications.[5] This is likely secondary to OSA patients often sleep deprived preoperatively, either secondary to anxiety or poor CPAP compliance.[37] Several studies have shown perioperative use of CPAP to have beneficial effects on reducing postoperative adverse events,[5,38,39] including reduced pain perception,[40,41] ultimately resulting in a decreased need for postoperative analgesics and fewer episodes of respiratory depression. Therefore, whenever possible, patients should be asked to use CPAP before surgery.

Reflux and Aspiration Precautions

A substantial percentage of obese patients have OSA. Obese patients are at higher risk of gastroesophageal reflux[42] and aspiration during general anesthesia.[43] To reduce these risks, if planning a general anesthetic with a protected airway, obese patients should receive prophylaxis for reflux (H$_2$ blocker, proton pump inhibitor, or esophageal motility stimulant) prior to intubation.[44] There currently are no guidelines on reducing the risk of aspiration for nonintubated OSA patients receiving intravenous (IV) sedation in an ambulatory setting, but similar measures should be considered.

INTRAOPERATIVE MANAGEMENT
Obstructive Sleep Apnea and Anesthesia

Local anesthesia carries the lowest overall risk of complications for OSA patients. Choosing to provide typical outpatient IV sedation practiced by most oral and maxillofacial surgeons involves the preservation of spontaneous ventilation with an unsecured airway. As a result, the greatest concern is that of possible hypoventilation secondary to upper airway obstruction, resulting in hypoxemia and hypercarbia. Patients with OSA have increased sensitivity to the respiratory depressant effects of anesthetic agents,[45] including a decrease in upper airway dilator muscle activity and thereby increased upper airway collapsibility, resulting in an increased risk of obstructive events and subsequent hypoxemia.[46–48] Narcotics suppress respiratory drive, blunt the arousal response, and may lead to life-threatening hypoxemia.[49] Benzodiazepines similarly reduce upper airway dilator muscle tone and worsen sleep-disordered breathing.[50] Increasing the depth of propofol anesthesia is associated with a progressive increase in critical airway pressure and upper airway collapsibility.[48] Titrating the amount of sedatives and narcotics to the lowest possible dose while still providing an adequate level of sedation, without compromising ventilation, can be challenging to even the most experienced clinician. There may be obstruction and hypoventilation even with minimal administered anesthetic dosages. IV anesthetic agent selection for OSA patients generally includes the use of short-acting benzodiazepines or short-acting narcotics and avoidance of any long-acting sedative hypnotics, thus minimizing the risk of airway obstruction and hypoventilation. Simple mechanical relief of airway obstruction by a jaw thrust or chin lift often proves ineffective in OSA patients. An astute and experienced clinician has appropriate airway adjuncts readily available, including oropharyngeal/nasopharyngeal airways, laryngeal mask airways, Combitubes, videolaryngoscope, and so forth. Clinicians must always be prepared and equipped to provide a secure airway, fully recognizing that OSA patients typically have more difficult intubation than the general population. Often, general anesthesia with a secure airway is preferable to deep sedation without a secure airway, particularly for procedures that may mechanically compromise the airway. Outpatient general anesthesia is a viable option in this patient population, largely depending on consideration of a patient's OSA severity, associated comorbidities, and the type of anesthetic agents used that may require prolonged postoperative monitoring.

POSTOPERATIVE MANAGEMENT

Organizations (ASA and Society for Ambulatory Anesthesia) have provided updated guidelines for the perioperative management of OSA patients,[22,51] but acknowledge that most recommendations are based on lower levels of evidence. Unfortunately, limited literature exists for evaluating the risks for typical outpatient oral and maxillofacial surgery patients. Several studies from the orthopedic, general, and other surgical services have shown increased risks for postoperative respiratory, pulmonary, and cardiovascular complications in an OSA population.[5–7,52] In the largest study to date, Memtsoudis and colleagues[6] examined more than 3 million records of US patients undergoing general and orthopedic surgery (ie, total knee and hip arthroplasty) and found that OSA is an independent risk factor for postoperative pulmonary complications. In a follow-up study, Memtsoudis and colleagues[18] found a lower incidence of postoperative complications among an OSA population involving more than 40,000 patients, with the use of neuraxial anesthesia compared with general anesthesia. Such a study, involving typical monitored anesthesia care in combination with neuraxial anesthesia, should correlate closely with typical outpatient IV sedation as practiced by most oral and maxillofacial surgeons.

Rapid Eye Movement Sleep Rebound

Anesthesia results in highly fragmented sleep during the first 2 postoperative nights, resulting in a significant reduction in rapid eye movement (REM) sleep.[53,54] In addition, opioids have been found to suppress REM sleep, while increasing the severity and duration of hypoxemia and central apneas.[5,55] Initial REM sleep suppression, however, is followed by REM sleep rebound approximately 3 to 5 days after surgery, resulting in possible worsening of obstructive symptoms. Older patients with more severe preoperative OSA and higher postoperative opioid requirements have more obstructive events postoperatively.[54]

To manage the increased AHI typically seen postoperatively in OSA patients, postoperative CPAP use has been extensively investigated. A recent matched cohort study[39] of 20,488 patients found a significantly increased risk of respiratory and cardiovascular complications when CPAP was not used postoperatively by patients with OSA. In addition, those patients with OSA using CPAP postoperatively had a risk of postoperative cardiovascular complications less than half those

with undiagnosed OSA.[39] Most importantly, only patients with severe or undiagnosed OSA not using CPAP postoperatively had a significantly increased risk of respiratory and cardiovascular complications. This is the first study to show a positive association between the severity of OSA and postoperative risks.[39]

Postoperative Medications

All opiates cause dose-dependent respiratory depression and resultant hypoventilation, hypoxia, and hypercarbia. The effects are exacerbated in OSA patients, with potentially fatal results. As a result, the foundation of postoperative analgesia should come from the use of nonsteroidal

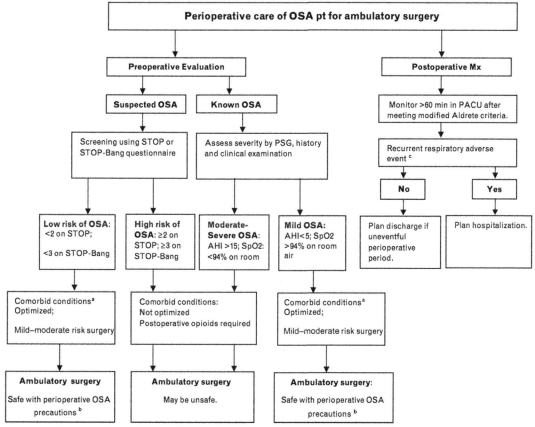

Fig. 1. Flowchart showing perioperative management of OSA patient undergoing ambulatory surgery. [a] Comorbid conditions: obesity (BMI >35 kg/m²), metabolic syndrome, cerebrovascular disease, uncontrolled hypertension, arrythmias, and heart failure. [b] Perioperative OSA precautions: anticipate possible difficult airway, short-acting anesthetic medications, ensure adequate reversal of neuromuscular blockade, extubate in head-up position. [c] Recurrent respiratory adverse event: any event occurring more than once in each 30-minute evaluation period. It includes 1 of the following events: oxygen saturation less than 90% on nasal cannula (3 episodes), hypopnea less than 8/min (3 episodes), apnea more than 10 seconds (1 episode), pain sedation mismatches (high pain and sedation scores concurrently).[59] Mx, management; PACU, postanesthetic care unit. (*From* Ankichetty S, Chung F. Considerations for patients with obstructive sleep apnea undergoing ambulatory surgery. Curr Opin Anaesthesiol 2011;24(6):608; with permission.)

anti-inflammatory agents (ibuprofen, ketorolac, naproxen, and celecoxib), acetaminophen or the centrally acting agents, such as tramadol hydrochloride. The concomitant use of narcotic agents should be titrated for pain severity and used only when nonnarcotic agents prove ineffective.[56] Stronger narcotic agents should be used only when weaker analgesic agents are not adequate. Mild to moderate pain can be treated with oral opioid agents, such as codeine, hydrocodone, oxycodone, and propoxyphene, because these agents have only mild effects on the respiratory system. Sedating antiemetics should be avoided because they may contribute to postoperative airway obstruction.

Criteria for Discharge

Patients with mild to moderate OSA whose comorbid conditions have been optimized should be able to safely undergo outpatient surgery. Those patients with severe OSA, whose comorbid conditions have not been optimized and require postoperative opioids, should not be considered for outpatient surgery[57] (**Fig. 1**). A study[58] evaluating otolaryngology patients undergoing combined nasal and palatal surgery used the following criteria for same-day discharge: (1) sustained O_2 saturation of 94% or greater on room air while asleep, (2) no history of cardiopulmonary disease or diabetes mellitus, (3) adequate oral analgesia and oral intake, (4) hemostasis, and (5) normal vital signs. The investigators found no postoperative complications in those patients discharged home the same day as surgery. Current ASA guidelines[22] recommend that patients at increased perioperative risk from OSA should only be discharged home when they are no longer at risk of postoperative respiratory depression. Moreover, patients must be able to maintain adequate oxygenation while breathing room air in an unstimulated environment. Ideally, patients should be monitored, preferably while asleep, on room air to ensure adequate oxygenation prior to discharge home. The suggested length of monitoring depends on the OSA severity, type and amount of anesthetic agents used, and patient comorbidities but should be for a minimum of 1 hour in an undisturbed state breathing room air. Clinicians should be guided by a patient's clinical picture. If a patient has questionable apneic episodes in the first hour, further monitoring is necessary until cardiovascular and respiratory status stabilizes. All patients must be reminded to always uses CPAP postoperatively, even for a brief rest, during the first postoperative week.

SUMMARY

Ambulatory surgery has historically been considered a safe and efficient option for appropriately selected patients. By carefully selecting patients based on their OSA severity and comorbidities, many patients with OSA can safely undergo surgical procedures on an outpatient basis. The severity of a patient's OSA, the invasiveness of the procedure, and the requirement for postoperative analgesics, however, should be taken into account when determining whether patients are at increased perioperative risk from their OSA.

REFERENCES

1. Nieto FJ, Young TB, Lind BK, et al. Association of sleep-disordered breathing, sleep apnea, and hypertension in a large community-based study. Sleep Heart Health Study. JAMA 2000;283(14):1829–36.
2. Hoyer FF, Lickfett LM, Mittmann-Braun E, et al. High prevalence of obstructive sleep apnea in patients with resistant paroxysmal atrial fibrillation after pulmonary vein isolation. J Interv Card Electrophysiol 2010;29(1):37–41.
3. Young T, Peppard PE, Gottlieb DJ. Epidemiology of obstructive sleep apnea: a population health perspective. Am J Respir Crit Care Med 2002; 165(9):1217–39.
4. Chung SA, Yuan H, Chung F. A systemic review of obstructive sleep apnea and its implications for anesthesiologists. Anesth Analg 2008;107(5):1543–63.
5. Gupta RM, Parvizi J, Hanssen AD, et al. Postoperative complications in patients with obstructive sleep apnea syndrome undergoing hip or knee replacement: a case-control study. Mayo Clin Proc 2001; 76(9):897–905.
6. Memtsoudis S, Liu SS, Ma Y, et al. Perioperative pulmonary outcomes in patients with sleep apnea after noncardiac surgery. Anesth Analg 2011; 112(1):113–21.
7. Vasu TS, Doghramji K, Cavallazzi R, et al. Obstructive sleep apnea syndrome and postoperative complications: clinical use of the STOP-BANG questionnaire. Arch Otolaryngol Head Neck Surg 2010;136(10):1020–4.
8. Young T, Palta M, Dempsey J, et al. The occurrence of sleep-disordered breathing among middle-aged adults. N Engl J Med 1993;328(17):1230–5.
9. Peppard PE, Young T, Barnet JH, et al. Increased prevalence of sleep-disordered breathing in adults. Am J Epidemiol 2013;177(9):1006–14.
10. Kim JA, Lee JJ. Preoperative predictors of difficult intubation in patients with obstructive sleep apnea syndrome. Can J Anaesth 2006;53(4):393–7.
11. Marshall NS, Wong KKH, Cullen SRJ, et al. Sleep apnea and 20-year follow-up for all-cause mortality,

stroke, and cancer incidence and mortality in the Busselton Health Study cohort. J Clin Sleep Med 2014;10(4):355–62.

12. Logan AG, Perlikowski SM, Mente A, et al. High prevalence of unrecognized sleep apnoea in drug-resistant hypertension. J Hypertens 2001;19(12): 2271–7.

13. Einhorn D, Stewart DA, Erman MK, et al. Prevalence of sleep apnea in a population of adults with type 2 diabetes mellitus. Endocr Pract 2007;13(4):355–62.

14. Gami AS, Pressman G, Caples SM, et al. Association of atrial fibrillation and obstructive sleep apnea. Circulation 2004;110(4):364–7.

15. O'Keeffe T, Patterson EJ. Evidence supporting routine polysomnography before bariatric surgery. Obes Surg 2004;14(1):23–6.

16. Schäfer H, Koehler U, Ewig S, et al. Obstructive sleep apnea as a risk marker in coronary artery disease. Cardiology 1999;92(2):79–84.

17. Basoglu OK, Vardar R, Tasbakan MS, et al. Obstructive sleep apnea syndrome and gastroesophageal reflux disease: the importance of obesity and gender. Sleep Breath 2015;19(2):585–92.

18. Memtsoudis SG, Stundner O, Rasul R, et al. Sleep apnea and total joint arthroplasty under various types of anesthesia: a population-based study of perioperative outcomes. Reg Anesth Pain Med 2013;38(4):274–81.

19. Oldenburg O, Lamp B, Faber L, et al. Sleep-disordered breathing in patients with symptomatic heart failure: a contemporary study of prevalence in and characteristics of 700 patients. Eur J Heart Fail 2007;9(3):251–7.

20. Garrigue S, Pépin J-L, Defaye P, et al. High prevalence of sleep apnea syndrome in patients with long-term pacing: the European Multicenter Polysomnographic Study. Circulation 2007;115(13): 1703–9.

21. Frey WC, Pilcher J. Obstructive sleep-related breathing disorders in patients evaluated for bariatric surgery. Obes Surg 2003;13(5):676–83.

22. American Society of Anesthesiologists Task Force on Perioperative Management of Patients with Obstructive Sleep Apnea. Practice guidelines for the perioperative management of patients with obstructive sleep apnea: an updated report by the American Society of Anesthesiologists Task Force on Perioperative Management of patients with obstructive sleep apnea. Anesthesiology 2014; 120(2):268–86.

23. Chung F, Yegneswaran B, Liao P, et al. STOP questionnaire: a tool to screen patients for obstructive sleep apnea. Anesthesiology 2008;108(5):812–21.

24. Finkel KJ, Searleman AC, Tymkew H, et al. Prevalence of undiagnosed obstructive sleep apnea among adult surgical patients in an academic medical center. Sleep Med 2009;10(7):753–8.

25. Singh M, Liao P, Kobah S, et al. Proportion of surgical patients with undiagnosed obstructive sleep apnoea. Br J Anaesth 2013;110(4):629–36.

26. Young T, Finn L, Peppard PE, et al. Sleep disordered breathing and mortality: eighteen-year follow-up of the Wisconsin sleep cohort. Giles T. Sleep 2008; 31(8):1071–8.

27. Fava C, Montagnana M, Favaloro E, et al. Obstructive sleep apnea syndrome and cardiovascular diseases. Semin Thromb Hemost 2011;37(03):280–97.

28. Al Lawati NM, Patel SR, Ayas NT. Epidemiology, risk factors, and consequences of obstructive sleep apnea and short sleep duration. Prog Cardiovasc Dis 2009;51(4):285–93.

29. Gami AS, Olson EJ, Shen WK, et al. Obstructive sleep apnea and the risk of sudden cardiac death: a longitudinal study of 10,701 adults. J Am Coll Cardiol 2013;62(7):610–6.

30. Iber C. The AASM Manual for the Scoring of Sleep and Associated Events. Darien (IL): American Academy of Sleep Medicine; 2007.

31. Collop NA, Anderson WM, Boehlecke B, et al. Clinical guidelines for the use of unattended portable monitors in the diagnosis of obstructive sleep apnea in adult patients. Portable monitoring task force of the American Academy of Sleep Medicine. J Clin Sleep Med 2007;3(7):737–47.

32. Chung F, Nagappa M, Singh M, et al. CPAP in the perioperative setting: evidence of support. Chest 2016;149(2):586–97.

33. Mehta V, Subramanyam R, Shapiro CM, et al. Health effects of identifying patients with undiagnosed obstructive sleep apnea in the preoperative clinic: a follow-up study. Can J Anaesth 2012; 59(6):544–55.

34. Cooksey JA, Balachandran JS. Portable monitoring for the diagnosis of OSA. Chest 2016; 149(4):1074–81.

35. Zonato AI, Martinho FL, Bittencourt LR, et al. Head and neck physical examination: comparison between nonapneic and obstructive sleep apnea patients. Laryngoscope 2005;115(6):1030–4.

36. Schwartz RN, Payne RJ, Forest V-I, et al. The relationship between upper airway collapse and the severity of obstructive sleep apnea syndrome: a chart review. J Otolaryngol Head Neck Surg 2015;44(1):32.

37. Aurell J, Elmqvist D. Sleep in the surgical intensive care unit: continuous polygraphic recording of sleep in nine patients receiving postoperative care. Br Med J (Clin Res Ed) 1985;290(6474):1029–32.

38. Liao P, Yegneswaran B, Vairavanathan S, et al. Postoperative complications in patients with obstructive sleep apnea: a retrospective matched cohort study. Can J Anaesth 2009;56(11):819–28.

39. Mutter TC, Chateau D, Moffatt M, et al. A matched cohort study of postoperative outcomes in obstructive sleep apnea: could preoperative diagnosis

and treatment prevent complications? Anesthesiology 2014;121(4):707–18.

40. Khalid I, Roehrs TA, Hudgel DW, et al. Continuous positive airway pressure in severe obstructive sleep apnea reduces pain sensitivity. Sleep 2011;34(12):1687–91.

41. Onen SH, Onen F, Albrand G, et al. Pain tolerance and obstructive sleep apnea in the elderly. J Am Med Dir Assoc 2010;11(9):612–6.

42. Demeester TR, Johnson LF, Joseph GJ, et al. Patterns of gastroesophageal reflux in health and disease. Ann Surg 1976;184(4):459–70.

43. Vaughan RW, Bauer S, Wise L. Volume and pH of gastric juice in obese patients. Anesthesiology 1975;43(6):686–9.

44. Warwick JP, Mason DG. Obstructive sleep apnoea syndrome in children. Anaesthesia 1998;53(6):571–9.

45. Chung F, Ankichetty S, Wong J. A systematic review of the effects of sedatives and anesthetics in patients with obstructive sleep apnea. J Anaesthesiol Clin Pharmacol 2011;27(4):447–58.

46. Drummond GB. Comparison of sedation with midazolam and ketamine: effects on airway muscle activity. Br J Anaesth 1996;76(5):663–7.

47. Drummond G. Influence of thiopentone on upper airway muscles. Br J Anaesth 1989;63(1):12–21.

48. Eastwood PR, Platt PR, Shepherd K, et al. Collapsibility of the upper airway at different concentrations of propofol anesthesia. Anesthesiology 2005;103(3):470–7.

49. Hillman DR, Eastwood PR. Upper airway, obstructive sleep apnea, and anesthesia. Sleep Med Clin 2013;8(1):23–8.

50. Guilleminault C, Silvestri R, Mondini S, et al. Aging and sleep apnea: action of benzodiazepine, acetazolamide, alcohol, and sleep deprivation in a healthy elderly group. J Gerontol 1984;39(6):655–61.

51. Joshi GP, Ankichetty SP, Gan TJ, et al. Society for Ambulatory Anesthesia consensus statement on preoperative selection of adult patients with obstructive sleep apnea scheduled for ambulatory surgery. Anesth Analg 2012;115(5):1060–8.

52. Gali B, Whalen FX, Schroeder DR, et al. Identification of patients at risk for postoperative respiratory complications using a preoperative obstructive sleep apnea screening tool and postanesthesia care assessment. Anesthesiology 2009;110(4):869–77.

53. Ellis BW, Dudley HAF. Some aspects of sleep research in surgical stress. J Psychosom Res 1976;20(4):303–8.

54. Rosenberg-Adamsen S, Skarbye M, Wildschiødtz G, et al. Sleep after laparoscopic cholecystectomy. Br J Anaesth 1996;77(5):572–5.

55. Bernards CM, Knowlton SL, Schmidt DF, et al. Respiratory and sleep effects of remifentanil in volunteers with moderate obstructive sleep apnea. Anesthesiology 2009;110(1):41–9.

56. Johnson QL, Netzer A. Opiate analgesics and the perioperative management of patients with obstructive sleep apnea. Mol Med 2015;112(6):435–8.

57. Ankichetty S, Chung F. Considerations for patients with obstructive sleep apnea undergoing ambulatory surgery. Curr Opin Anaesthesiol 2011;24(6):605–11.

58. Kieff DA, Busaba NY. Same-day discharge for selected patients undergoing combined nasal and palatal surgery for obstructive sleep apnea. Ann Otol Rhinol Laryngol 2004;113(2):128–31.

59. Seet E, Chung F. Obstructive sleep apnea: preoperative assessment. Anesthesiol Clin 2010;28:199–215.

Discharge Criteria, Impact of the Patient and the Procedure

What the Oral Surgeon Should Know

Kyle J. Kramer, DDS, MS

KEYWORDS

- Discharge criteria • Anesthesia • PONV • Recovery

KEY POINTS

- There is a definite need for the use of objective criteria to assist with assessment of a patient deemed ready for discharge.
- The use of a standardized discharge criteria checklist is recommended but must be further individualized for each patient.
- The development of a rational plan for postoperative pain management and prevention/management of postoperative nausea and vomiting is essential for success.
- A thorough understanding of the pharmacodynamics and pharmacokinetics of medications administered is crucial for patient safety.
- Early identification of potential problems and proper intervention help minimize patient risk.

GENERAL OVERVIEW OF DISCHARGE CRITERIA

Although the intraoperative periods involving the delivery of local anesthesia as well as the completion of the surgical procedure itself remain the most likely times requiring emergency intervention, the recovery or immediate postoperative period is also of key importance.[1] In fact, one of the weakest links regarding patient safety for sedation and anesthesia in the dental ambulatory setting is determining when the patient can safely be discharged from supervised care. This is mainly due to the patient transitioning from a highly supervised area, where the clinician can easily identify potential complications and provide early intervention, to areas in which the patient is far removed from skilled care, such as their home or automobile. It is precisely because of these concerns that the clinician must use the utmost care and skill in identifying which patients are ready for discharge and those who require additional monitored time to recover. In 2002, the American Society of Anesthesiologists published guidelines for the use of sedation and anesthesia by nonanesthesiologists that detail recovery parameters and discharge criteria.[2] Furthermore, specific criteria regarding the recovery and discharge of dental patients undergoing sedation and anesthesia have been published by the American Dental Association and the American Association of Oral and Maxillofacial Surgeons.[3–5] Ideally, this decision-making process should include not only the practitioner's own professional judgment, but also a system using clear, objective findings. There have been several systems developed to assist with this task, such as the Glasgow Coma Scale, Aldrete and Modified Aldrete Score, Postanesthesia Discharge Scoring System (PADSS), Pediatric Discharge Scoring System (Ped-PADSS), and the Postoperative Quality Recovery Scale.[6–8] Although the final decision to discharge a patient

Department of Oral Surgery and Hospital Dentistry, Indiana University School of Dentistry, 550 University Boulevard, Room 3195, Indianapolis, IN 46202, USA
E-mail address: kjkramer@iu.edu

Oral Maxillofacial Surg Clin N Am 29 (2017) 197–208
http://dx.doi.org/10.1016/j.coms.2016.12.009
1042-3699/17/© 2017 Elsevier Inc. All rights reserved.

always remains with the individual clinician, any and all auxiliary support staff should be encouraged to notify the practitioner of any concerns or questions they have regarding the stability of the patient's recovery. A systematic approach, which will be discussed in further detail, provides built-in redundancies that help prevent a patient from being discharged from the dental ambulatory setting prematurely, thereby helping reduce the likelihood of an emergency arising that cannot be easily treated by the practitioner.

STANDARD DISCHARGE CRITERIA

A crucial aspect of a comprehensive, time-based anesthetic record should include a section covering the recovery period as well as identification of a standardized set of discharge criteria that must be documented before the patient's discharge. These discharge criteria are detailed in **Box 1**. It is of key importance to understand that these criteria, although standardized, must be altered when necessary based on the patient's medical comorbidities, the surgical intervention, and the anesthetic management. It is the clinician's responsibility to identify potential concerns, adjust the standardized criteria when necessary, and document these changes once the patient fulfills them satisfactorily. An example of an alteration may include a pulse oximetry reading of 95% on 1 L of oxygen, which mirrors the patient's baseline preoperative state.

Ideally, part of any standardized anesthetic record should incorporate a section covering the immediate postoperative period, including the full extent of the recovery time before discharge. Many records use checkoff boxes that specifically state the criteria listed in **Box 1** to help prevent

accidentally omitting a key component. The record also should include the actual time the patient was deemed ready for discharge from the office in addition to the actual discharge time, if there was any difference due to a non–medically related delay. If a delay was due to an unforeseen medically related issue, necessitating further monitoring and/or care, the record should be amended as such. Finally, the discharge section also should include a note indicating in whose care the patient was discharged from the office.

REVIEW OF SPECIFIC DISCHARGE CRITERIA
Level of Consciousness

The patient's level of consciousness following the delivery of any sedatives or anesthetics must return to their baseline or preoperative state before discharge home. Recovery times can vary significantly between patients and even between appointments for the same patient, depending on the specifics of the anesthetic and surgical plan. The patient should remain in the treatment area under the immediate supervision and monitored care of the anesthesia provider until consciousness has been regained. Then, assuming the patient is otherwise stable, the patient may be safely transported to an alternative recovery area under the immediate monitored care of trained staff if desired. Many dental offices lack a separate dedicated recovery or postanesthesia care unit area and elect instead to recover and discharge the patient directly from the treatment area/operatory. The surgeon or anesthesia provider must remain on the premises until the patient is discharged in case immediate intervention is required.

The timing of when the intravenous catheter (IV) should be discontinued remains somewhat controversial. Some practitioners elect to remove the IV catheter early after emergence from sedation or anesthesia, mainly for pediatric patients. The main reasons for discontinuing the IV so early is to help calm the patient and/or parents and to minimize discomfort associated with the removal of the IV catheter. However, this practice is not highly recommended, because an unforeseen complication occurring after removal of the IV catheter may require subsequent cannulation attempts to enable appropriate patient management. This may become a highly difficult or impossible task to complete in a timely manner if the patient is uncooperative or has poor venous access, thereby possibly compromising an effective response. Far more often, the risk-benefit analysis tends to favor maintaining IV access throughout the recovery period. The vast majority

---

Box 1
Standard discharge criteria checklist

☐ Awake, responsive, and oriented

☐ Minimal/no postoperative nausea and vomiting

☐ Instructions discussed: escort/patient

☐ Received written postoperative instructions

☐ Heart rate and blood pressure within 20% of baseline

☐ SpO$_2$ >90%

☐ Postoperative pain controlled

☐ All questions answered before discharge

☐ Patient discharged from clinic in care of:

_____

of patients, both adult and pediatric, are typically able to tolerate the IV catheter with minimal to no distress. Additionally, continued IV access permits immediate IV access for emergencies or complications without necessitating another "stick." Practically speaking, the removal of the catheter itself can be done in a minimally stimulating way, helping to reduce patient distress.

Patients who are recovering from the effects of administered sedatives and anesthetic agents should be permitted to rest quietly while the drugs are redistributed, metabolized, and eliminated, as these processes simply take time. The anesthesia provider must ensure the peak effect of any drug administered has occurred before the patient is cleared for discharge. Otherwise the risk of deleterious effects occurring outside the monitored care setting increases significantly. Anesthesia providers must consider the pharmacokinetic profile of a sedative or anesthetic drug when selecting appropriate agents and techniques. Anesthetic drug options with very short redistribution or elimination half-lives tend to be more ideal than agents with prolonged clinical profiles when taking the recovery period into consideration.

It is not advisable to routinely administer reversal agents simply for the purpose of facilitating a more rapid emergence and recovery, even when possible. Although this may be a tempting strategy, it is fraught with unnecessary and potentially life-threatening risk. A review of the pharmacokinetic profile for flumazenil easily demonstrates the risk of routine reversal of benzodiazepines. Flumazenil has a relatively short terminal half-life (40–80 minutes).[9] This creates a potential risk for resedation after the antagonistic effects of flumazenil wane if used to reverse benzodiazepines with longer redistribution and terminal half-lives.[10,11] If a patient is given flumazenil to promote a rapid emergence and then subsequently discharged, the patient may become resedated at home. This is clearly problematic should a complication necessitating intervention arise. A similar phenomenon can be applied equally to opioid antagonists, such as naloxone. As such, reversal agents, such as flumazenil or naloxone should be reserved for situations necessitating emergent or urgent antagonistic activity only. These reversal drugs necessitate a prolonged monitoring period of typically 2 hours when used in these types of situations to properly ensure resedation does not occur.

Stability of Vital Signs: Ventilation

The overwhelming majority of complications or emergencies for patients receiving sedation or anesthesia for dental procedures are related to disruptions in normal respiratory functionality.[12–15] With this in mind, clinicians must be overtly aware of and continuously monitor the patient's ability to exchange air and maintain adequate oxygenation. One common example would be a patient who begins to exhibit obstruction due to relaxation of the musculature of the upper airway once sedated.[16] Equally important as stability of oxygenation is the patient's ability to maintain adequate ventilation. Ventilation can be assessed in a multitude of ways, such as visually monitoring the patient's breathing excursions (chest and abdominal wall movements) in combination with precordial/pretracheal auscultation and capnography.[17] Ideally, all of these options should be used in concert, with the goal of ensuring the patient continues to exchange air without interruption.[18] The use of nasal cannulas that simultaneously deliver supplemental oxygen while also sampling for gas analysis (ie, capnography) are ideal for dental patients, as they do not impair access to the oral cavity.

During the recovery period, patients must be continuously monitored for signs of impaired ventilation. This is easily facilitated by continuous monitoring via capnography in combination with pretracheal auscultation. Once the patient emerges from sedation or anesthesia, the amount of supplemental oxygen can be titrated slowly off. The nasal cannula system, however, will permit continued ventilatory monitoring that the patient is likely to tolerate well. If a nasopharyngeal airway (NPA) was placed to help facilitate air exchange, it can be removed easily and with minimal discomfort once the patient is awake. There should be no rush to remove the NPA earlier, as patients can easily tolerate an NPA, even when awake. Use of lidocaine ointment to facilitate easy placement of the NPA provides an added benefit by anesthetizing the mucosa, leading to improved patient tolerance of the airway adjunct. Also, postponed removal of the NPA will decrease the risk of laryngospasm should bleeding of the nasal mucosa occur.

Patients should remain in a monitored care setting until they have demonstrated ability to maintain adequate ventilation. Patients should be able to exchange air spontaneously, without any prompting or support and should have a respiratory rate within 20% of their baseline or preoperative value. Although a minimal or modest degree of respiratory depression is expected if the patient was given an opioid agonist, a respiratory rate below 8 breaths per minute warrants further monitoring and potential intervention.

Stability of Vital Signs: Oxygenation

Assessment of the patient's ability to maintain adequate oxygenation must occur before discharge. It is strongly recommended that the patient's oxygenation be continuously monitored throughout the entirety of the recovery period. This is easily accomplished using a noninvasive pulse oximeter. The patient should be able to maintain pulse oximeter values approximating those noted preoperatively. Clinicians must be cognizant regarding the use of supplemental oxygen when assessing preoperative and postoperative values. If no supplemental oxygen was delivered when the preoperative assessment was taken, then the patient should be able to maintain similar values postoperatively on room air alone before discharge. Those who normally require supplemental oxygen, such as patients with chronic obstructive pulmonary disease, must be assessed using the same degree of oxygen augmentation as before discharge. Care also must be taken to ensure the stability of the patient's oxygenation was assessed after enough time had passed following the cessation of supplemental oxygen so as to prevent artificially elevated readings that are likely to drop precipitously shortly thereafter. A period of 5 to 10 minutes on room air with a pulse oximeter reading approximating the preoperative baseline is generally considered acceptable. Patients who have pulse oximeter readings at or below 95% should be promptly evaluated and are likely unsuitable for discharge home.

Stability of Vital Signs: Circulation

Before discharge, patients should be continuously monitored for acute changes involving their cardiovascular system, most commonly their blood pressure and heart rate. Most of the commonly used anesthetic agents are associated with the potential for causing hypotension and bradycardia. However, some patients may experience hypertension and/or tachycardia, possibly due to inadequate analgesia postoperatively. As such, clinicians must be acutely aware of the patient's "normal" preoperative blood pressure and heart rate, able to identify concerning cardiovascular trends, and be ready to intervene accordingly. Patients demonstrating mild to modest depression of their cardiovascular system often respond well to basic measures, such as fluid boluses, and administration of short-acting vasopressors, such as ephedrine or phenylephrine. Initial steps for patients trending in the opposite direction should include assessment for adequate analgesia before cardiovascular pharmacologic intervention, such as beta blockers or other antihypertensive agents.

Similar to other vital signs, the patient should remain in a monitored care setting until cleared for discharge and should be within 20% of their preoperative cardiovascular baseline values. Assessment and documentation of the trends throughout the entirety of the recovery period is crucial. It is generally recommended the sphygmomanometer and electrocardiogram (ECG) remain in place until the patient is deemed stable and ready to leave. This typically is not a concern, as patients usually tolerate ECG pads and a noninvasive blood pressure cuff without difficulty.

Stability of Vital Signs: Temperature

Oral surgical patients receiving sedation and anesthesia using agents aside from those that are a risk for triggering malignant hyperthermia (volatile agents, succinylcholine) may not necessarily require monitoring perioperatively with regard to temperature. However, there may be specific circumstances in which monitoring the patient's temperature perioperatively would be indicated. For example, patients who present with infections and may be at risk for sepsis are likely to benefit from this type of monitoring. Additionally, patients who receive inhalational anesthetic agents, such as sevoflurane, should be monitored as such perioperatively.[5] A rise in temperature (>38.8°C; 101.8°F) due to the development of a hypermetabolic state is a late but critical sign of malignant hyperthermia.[19] It is possible this may be seen during recovery or even well beyond discharge of the patient. As such, patients should not only be monitored accordingly during the perioperative period, but also should receive postoperative instructions regarding development of a postoperative fever. Aside from these rare clinical outliers, patients can be safely discharged once their temperature approximates their preoperative baseline value. A modest decrease in body temperature while under general anesthesia is expected due to impairment of the body's normal thermoregulatory processes, as well as the vasodilatory activity of most anesthetic agents.[20] This commonly triggers some mild shivering during recovery that passes with the tincture of time.[21] Other patient comfort strategies include use of blankets and layered clothing, as well as forced air warmer systems.[22,23]

Control of Bleeding

Some degree of postoperative bleeding is common following most invasive oral surgical procedures. Patients should be assessed for adequacy of hemostasis before discharge. Any patient who continues to actively bleed should not be discharged until the bleeding can be stopped. Additionally, it is crucial to discuss proper hemostasis basics with patients and their escorts. For most dentoalveolar surgical procedures, this typically includes use of and instructions for changing gauze pressure dressings. If the surgical procedure necessitates special or alternative dressings, patients should receive the instructions preoperatively, if possible, and then review them once again before discharge. Of particular note for oral surgeons is the use of small gauze dressings, such as 2 × 2 gauze pads. These small gauze dressings, especially if not ligated together with floss, become an aspiration risk when placed posteriorly as a surgical dressing, which is common following third molar extractions. In fact, there have been multiple instances of oral surgical and dental patients who suffered significant morbidity and mortality after aspiration of small gauze or cotton rolls.

Control of Vomiting/Nausea

Postoperative nausea and vomiting (PONV) is a huge area of concern for any anesthesia provider due to the negative impact on the patient's experience. The risk of PONV is multifactorial, as seen in **Boxes 2–4**.[24–26] Anesthesia providers must weight patient, surgical, and anesthetic risk factors when deciding how best to prevent and manage PONV.[27] For dental ambulatory anesthesia, a rational preventive strategy includes a stepped approach based initially on the number of risk factors, as seen in **Table 1**. Patients with a low risk (0–1 risk factor) do not necessarily require preventive therapy and may be best managed using a "wait and see" approach to avoid rare but potentially significant side effects associated with some antiemetics. For patients with moderate risk (2–3 risk factors), selected use of 1 or 2 different modalities is often effective,

whereas 2 or more combined modalities are recommended for patients with high risk (4–5 risk factors).[27]

A common approach for oral surgical patients with moderate risk includes the administration of IV dexamethasone (0.1 mg/kg, up to 4 mg/kg) immediately following induction.[28–30] Dexamethasone is rather unique with regard to other corticosteroids and its antiemetic potential; however, the delayed onset requires early administration and renders it less useful as a rescue option.[31] Additionally, IV ondansetron (0.1 mg/kg, up to 4 mg/kg) can be administered toward the end of the case, ideally 15 to 30 minutes before emergence.[32] Patients who are experiencing uncontrolled PONV during the recovery period should not be discharged from the office until control is regained, which often requires prolonged time in the monitored care setting. Should the patient experience PONV during the recovery period, small, incremental boluses of diluted promethazine (6.125–12.5 mg for adults, up to 25 mg; 0.25–1 mg/kg for pediatric patients) can be slowly titrated to effect.[33,34] Sedation is an expected side effect of promethazine, somewhat similar to the

---

Box 3
Simplified postoperative nausea and vomiting risk factors for children

Surgery ≥30 minutes

Age ≥3 years

Strabismus surgery

History of postoperative nausea and vomiting in relatives

Data from Eberhart LH, Geldner G, Kranke P, et al. The development and validation of a risk score to predict the probability of postoperative vomiting in pediatric patients. Anesth Analg 2004;99(6):1630–7.

Box 2
Simplified postoperative nausea and vomiting risk factors for adults

Female gender

Nonsmoker

History of postoperative nausea and vomiting

Postoperative opioids

Data from Apfel CC, Laara E, Koivuranta M, et al. A simplified risk score for predicting postoperative nausea and vomiting: conclusions from cross-validations between two centers. Anesthesiology 1999;91(3):693–700.

Box 4
Simplified postdischarge nausea and vomiting risk factors for adults

Female gender

History of postoperative nausea and vomiting

Age younger than 50 years

Postoperative opioids

Nausea in postanesthesia care unit

Data from Apfel CC, Philip BK, Cakmakkaya OS, et al. Who is at risk for postdischarge nausea and vomiting after ambulatory surgery? Anesthesiology 2012;117(3):475–86.

Table 1
Severity of postoperative nausea and vomiting (PONV)/postdischarge nausea and vomiting (PDNV) risk

Total Number of Risk Factors	Severity of PONV/ PDNV Risk
0–1	Low risk
2–3	Moderate risk
>4	High risk

Data from Gan TJ, Diemunsch P, Habib AS, et al. Consensus guidelines for the management of postoperative nausea and vomiting. Anesth Analg 2014;118(1):85–113.

degree of sedation from diphenhydramine, which is likely to extend the recovery period. As such, administration of promethazine is recommended for rescue management and not for routine, prophylactic use.

With regard to antiemetic pharmacologic options, there are several generally accepted modalities, as seen in **Table 2**. Selection of any particular preventive modalities should include risk-benefit assessment for the patient, as well as cost-effectiveness analysis. Although the use of generic drug options can be beneficial in terms of selecting cheaper alternatives, the recent rash of various drug shortages has been somewhat problematic from a financial aspect. The anesthesia provider must be cognizant of the specifics (eg, dose, contraindications, potential side effects, drug interactions) regardless of the modality selected.

One particularly difficult situation that often faces oral surgeons and dental anesthesia providers is postdischarge nausea and vomiting (PDNV). Patients should be instructed to contact the practitioner should they begin to experience persistent or uncontrolled PDNV once released from the ambulatory dental setting. The practitioner is then faced with the decision of attempting to manage the PDNV remotely versus having the patient return either to the office or to the hospital for further evaluation and subsequent management. This decision must take into consideration a multitude of factors, such as the course of the surgical procedure, unanticipated perioperative complications, the patient's medical history, physical condition, and stability during the immediate recovery period, as well as the recovery at home based on the patient's verbal report. Clearly the patient should be personally evaluated if the practitioner determines there is a strong likelihood for further decline or compromise. Alternatively, for patients who are otherwise stable, 2 common strategies include use of ondansetron oral dissolving tablets (4–8 mg) or promethazine rectal suppositories (12.5–25 mg). Either option can be called into a local pharmacy and are very effective for managing otherwise uncomplicated PDNV.

Control of Postoperative Pain

Similar to the other vital signs, patients should remain under the direct care of the clinician until adequate pain control has occurred. There are several alternatives available for managing patients who are experiencing inadequate postoperative analgesia; however, some options are more ideal given the nature of the office-based dental ambulatory setting. The vast majority of office-based oral surgical procedures lend themselves well to the use of local anesthetics, which should be strongly considered as deemed appropriate. Bupivacaine is an excellent option, with its exceptionally prolonged duration of action, permitting time for other oral analgesics to act before the anesthetic effect waning.[35] Regardless of the means chosen, clinicians must ensure the patient has adequate pain control before discharge from the office.

Routine use of parenteral nonsteroidal anti-inflammatory drugs (NSAIDs), such as ketorolac remains somewhat controversial. Ketorolac has a rapid onset when administered intravenously and is an effective analgesic, anti-inflammatory, and antipyretic agent. It is rather popular for oral surgical procedures in the ambulatory setting and can be safely administered via IV to adult and pediatric patients (0.5–1 mg/kg, up to 30 mg total).[36–38] However, its use may be contraindicated, due to the impaired effect on platelet aggregation, based on the patient's comorbidities, concurrent medications, and, of course, the surgical procedure itself. When selected for use, care must be taken by the clinician to assess the patient after

Table 2
Antiemetic pharmacologic modalities

Drug Class	Generic Example(s)
5-HT$_3$ receptor antagonist	Ondansetron
NK-1 receptor antagonist	Aprepitant
Corticosteroid	Dexamethasone
Butyrophenone	Droperidol; Haloperidol
Antihistamine	Dimenhydrinate; Hydroxyzine
Anticholinergic	Scopolamine
Phenothiazine	Promethazine

administration for signs of prolonged or unusual bleeding. Patients also must be informed of when to begin their oral NSAIDs if parenteral NSAIDs are given, otherwise potential risk for overdose is established.

Opioid agonists, such as fentanyl, are a commonly used component of the sedative or anesthetic plan during the perioperative period. This group of analgesics is useful for blocking or impairing the upward flow of noxious stimuli from the periphery to the brain, which not only helps smooth out the course of the anesthetic, but also typically leads to a reduction in anesthetic requirements. Unfortunately, perioperative use of opioid agonists is strongly linked to an increased risk of PONV and PDNV.[27,39] Clinicians must balance the risk-benefit of avoiding the perioperative use of an opioid agonist as an effective means of reducing the risk of PONV and PDNV versus the strong analgesic potential that is associated with opioid use. Often using the minimal dose necessary during the perioperative period is a very effective means of managing the PONV/PDNV issue. Additionally, use of opioid agonists with shorter durations of action, such as fentanyl or alfentanil, can be beneficial, especially when combined with other analgesics, such as NSAIDs, acetaminophen, and local anesthetics, as the rapid redistribution and/or metabolism is likely to reduce the incidence of PDNV. For patients who continue to experience significant postoperative pain refractory to alternative means, opioids with longer durations of action, such as morphine or hydromorphone, are acceptable alternatives; however, patients are likely to benefit from prophylactic use of an appropriate antiemetic. Of these 2 particular agents, the pharmacokinetics of hydromorphone permit ease of titration, lessening the potential for accidental overdose and associated side effects.

The use of acetaminophen as a component for effective pain control during the postoperative period has long been a mainstay for oral surgery and dentistry. Acetaminophen is often combined with an opioid agonist and can be taken in conjunction with an NSAID to help maximize effective postoperative analgesia. With the approval of the Food and Drug Administration in 2010, the availability of IV acetaminophen (Ofirmev) permitted early administration before emergence, which not only helps increase analgesia during recovery but also can be useful for lowering opioid agonist requirements.[40] Currently, the main drawback for widespread use in oral surgery and dental anesthesia is mainly economical because IV acetaminophen is rather expensive. Simply put, the cost for IV acetaminophen is currently not practical for everyday use. This is likely to change once the patent for Ofirmev expires in 2017, after which a more affordable generic version may become available.

Postoperative Instructions

In the current litigation-prone climate, there is no shortage of required documentation for patients and the written postoperative instructions are no exception. Clinicians must be sure that each patient receives written postoperative instructions that detail not only the specifics for the surgical procedure, but also any concerns regarding the anesthetic plan. Written instructions for patients who receive sedation or anesthesia should include the topics shown in **Box 5**. Ideally, these instructions should be reviewed verbally with the patient and the patient's escort before the procedure, while the patient is free of the effects of any sedatives, and again immediately before discharge. Should any complications have arisen necessitating specific alterations or additions to the instructions, notes indicating such changes should be made on the postoperative instruction document and included in the patient's medical chart as well. Patients also should be given an emergency contact number so that they can quickly contact the practitioner should an issue arise after discharge from the office.

SPECIAL ANESTHETIC CONCERNS

Of key importance to any practitioner providing sedation or anesthesia is a keen understanding of the pharmacodynamics and pharmacokinetics of the drugs administered during the perioperative period. The practitioner must understand and appreciate when the peak clinical effects of the drugs administered are likely to occur based on the specifics of the situation (eg, presence of confounding medical comorbidities, surgical factors, complications). Also important is the anticipated duration of action of the various medications administered. Anesthesia providers must be cognizant of these points when selecting which

---

Box 5
Written instructions

Postsedation or anesthesia written instructions should include details regarding the following:

- Postoperative diet
- Postoperative medication(s)
- Activities to avoid
- Contact number for an emergency

sedative or anesthetic medications to use. With regard to safe discharge of a patient, improper agent selection, poor understanding, or lack of identification of the peak effect of a particular agent are potential problems that can lead to significant patient morbidity and mortality, especially if occurring outside of a monitored care area. For example, a patient who receives an IV bolus of fentanyl immediately before discharge from the office is at risk for significant respiratory depression once the maximal peak effect occurs 5 to 15 minutes later. For this reason, anesthesia providers must be sure that the peak effect of any drug administered has occurred before deeming the patient safe for discharge.

Ketamine

As a dissociative anesthetic, ketamine is known to produce a rather unique clinical sedation and anesthesia profile. Potential side effects commonly found with ketamine include nystagmus, diplopia, PONV, and emergence delirium or hallucinations.[21,41] The vast majority of these side effects tend to be dose dependent.[42,43] Anesthesia providers who choose to use ketamine should take appropriate preventive steps when possible, assess patients for these specific complications, and provide proper management. Patients given ketamine may require extended monitoring before recovering fully and being deemed ready for discharge.

Pharmacologic Options

There are many pharmacologic sedative and anesthetic options available with extremely favorable pharmacokinetic profiles that match well for use with dental ambulatory anesthesia. Some common examples include midazolam, fentanyl, and propofol. Most of these drugs have rather clean recovery profiles, either due to rapid drug metabolism coupled with inactive metabolic byproducts or to redistribution to inactive body compartments, either of which tend to help facilitate a cleaner, more rapid recovery and subsequent discharge. Drugs that have active metabolites (diazepam or meperidine) or those with prolonged durations of actions (morphine, lorazepam) tend to be potentially more problematic and may be less than ideal when compared with the cleaner and shorter-acting alternatives. These factors should be taken into consideration by the anesthesia provider when selecting the various sedatives and anesthetic drugs to be administered. Generally speaking, drugs with a shorter duration of action tend to be more preferable for the ambulatory dental anesthesia setting, as

patients can be safely discharged once the peak effect has been observed and they return to their preoperative baseline.

SPECIAL PATIENT CONCERNS
Diabetic Patients

Patients who present with diabetes mellitus type I or II warrant special consideration regarding assessment before discharge. Practitioners must be acutely aware of their potential for perioperative alterations in blood glucose. As such, it is critical to assess the patient's blood glucose not only during the preoperative period, but also intraoperatively and during recovery as well. Depending on the potential lability of the specific patient, intraoperative measurements may span 30 to 60 minutes.[44] If the surgical procedure is relatively short, intraoperative measurements may be unnecessary. However, assessment and documentation of the patient's blood glucose before discharge is critical regardless of the length of the procedure. This is not only useful for ideal patient care but also crucial for medical-legal purposes.

Obstructive Sleep Apnea

The diagnosis of obstructive sleep apnea (OSA) is becoming more prevalent within the United States, especially as obesity rates continue to climb. Recent estimations show roughly 26% of Americans ages 30 to 70 have OSA.[45] Patients with OSA are likely to be overly sensitive to the sedative and anesthetic drugs, highly likely to experience airway obstruction perioperatively, and also more at risk for respiratory depression when opioid agonists are used for postoperative analgesia.

Further complicating matters is that only 10% to 20% of those with OSA have been actually diagnosed via polysomnography[46]; however, there are several tools that can be used to help identify patients who are at risk of OSA. The STOP-BANG assessment tool, seen in **Table 3**, is commonly used, efficient, and effective.[44,47] Patients are scored according to their responses on the STOP-BANG questionnaire and then subsequently managed based on their risk. Strategies for managing patients with known or suspected OSA include minimizing or avoiding opioid agonists, reinforcing appropriate use of nonopioid analgesics, and encouraging use of a continuous positive airway pressure (CPAP) machine at home when possible. Patients with known OSA who have a CPAP machine should be instructed to bring their CPAP to the surgical appointment, as it may be useful during the recovery period. Patients with known or suspected OSA should not be discharged until they are no longer at risk for

Table 3
STOP-BANG questionnaire

Snoring	Do you snore loudly (loud enough to be heard through closed doors)?
Tired	Do you often feel tired, fatigued, or sleepy during the daytime?
Observed	Has anyone observed you stop breathing during your sleep?
Blood Pressure	Do you have or are you being treated for high blood pressure?
Body mass index (BMI)	BMI >35 mg/m^2?
Age	Age older than 50 y?
Neck circumference	Is your neck circumference >40 cm?
Gender	Are you a male?
STOP-BANG Score	**Obstructive Sleep Apnea (OSA) Risk Stratification**
<3	Low risk of OSA
3+	High risk of OSA

From Chung F, Yegneswaran B, Liao P, et al. STOP questionnaire: a tool to screen patients for obstructive sleep apnea. Anesthesiology 2008;108(5):821; with permission.

postoperative respiratory depression and demonstrate the ability to maintain satisfactory respiratory function undisturbed, without supplemental oxygen.[48]

Pediatric, Geriatric, and Special Needs Patients

These patient groups can often present difficulties regarding their perioperative care and subsequent safe discharge. Of utmost importance is ensuring they have returned to their preoperative baseline state before leaving the office. Patients who are deemed fit for discharge before returning to their baseline level of consciousness are at risk for significant complications. A study of postdischarge adverse events for pediatric dental patients receiving conscious sedation using a variety of oral agents reported 60.1% of patients slept during the car ride home and 21.4% of that group were difficult to arouse on arriving home.[49] These data suggest the potential for patients being discharged prematurely, as well as the use of less than ideal anesthetic drugs or techniques. Pediatric, geriatric, and special needs patients are more likely to lack the needed reserve to safely tolerate a significant postdischarge complication, should it occur. As such, anesthesia providers must ensure such a patient is never discharged still "asleep."

Clinicians also must ensure that the patient's escort, often the parent(s) or spouse, is able to safely transport the patient home from the office and also is capable of understanding and providing basic care once home.[50] A review of 118 adverse sedation events specifically discussed multiple incidents of pediatric patients being injured in car seats on the way home. The proposed mechanism of injury included patients who fell asleep, developing airway obstruction due to their head position and not being able to self-correct due to residual sedative drug effects.[12] Therefore, patients who are likely to require assistance while being transported home (pediatric or special needs patients) may benefit from the presence of 2 adult escorts.[51] This will permit one person to safely operate the automobile, while the other can tend to the patient as necessary. Although this practice is ideal, it is not always possible depending on the degree of family support for a particular patient. Often it is possible to identify such potential concerns during the consultation appointment and simply request that another capable adult be on hand to assist on the day of surgery. If the safety of the patient is in question, it is prudent for the clinician to insist that the patient remain in the office until alternative accommodations can be arranged.

SPECIFIC PROCEDURES

The list of procedures performed by oral and maxillofacial surgeons is rather extensive and ever growing. With regard to discharging a patient after a procedure, the oral surgeon should ensure the patient is stable and approximating their baseline preoperative presentation. The oral surgeon must ensure any specific concerns or postoperative instructions regarding the procedure are reviewed in detail and understood by the patient and/or escort before discharge. As the operating surgeon, patient safety is the primary concern. Patients must be informed to contact the oral surgeon immediately if they experience any untoward complications, such as significant edema, dyspnea, or dysphagia. Although a fully trained staff member may be acceptable to supervise the patient in recovery, the final assessment of the patient's stability before discharge should be performed by the surgeon and anesthesia provider when appropriate. Depending on the specific surgical procedure, that assessment may include items such as physical evaluation of the surgical site, verification of adequate hemostasis, and lack of significant or increasing edema.

POSTOPERATIVE CHECKUP

It is highly recommended that practitioners follow-up with patients within a reasonable time after surgery following discharge home to verify that the patient's postoperative course has remained event free. This is typically accomplished by contacting the patient via telephone in the evening on the day of surgery. Not only does this telephone call help demonstrate the continued delivery of high-quality care, but also provides the means for identifying additional potential complications that have yet to fully manifest. For example, a patient with new-onset minor dysphagia and edema following otherwise uncomplicated surgical extraction of third molars may not feel comfortable calling the doctor, but this potential complication may be easily identified during the evening postoperative call by the surgeon. Additionally, the surgeon can verify that any specific postoperative instructions have been followed by the patient during this conversation, such as a patient with diabetes mellitus type I verifying that his or her blood glucose that evening was within the normal range. Any significant findings discovered by the surgeon during this conversation should be included in the patient's medical chart as deemed worthy.

SUMMARY

The use of objective criteria to help establish when a patient is fit for discharge is a crucial tool for practitioners, in addition to their own subjective assessment and clinical intuition. The discharge criteria discussed are generally accepted for the vast majority of patients but should be tailored to each individual patient based on the surgical procedure and anesthetic plan. Use of a discharge criteria checklist is recommended, as it helps reduce the likelihood of accidentally missing a key component. Other important keys include use of written discharge instructions and means for patients to quickly contact their surgeon or anesthesia provider should they experience a complication after discharge. Following up with patients the evening after surgery is a highly

recommended patient management option as well. Strict adherence to these principles decreases the risk that patients may suffer significant postoperative morbidity or mortality.

REFERENCES

1. Chicka MC, Dembo JB, Mathu-Muju KR, et al. Adverse events during pediatric dental anesthesia and sedation: a review of closed malpractice insurance claims. Pediatr Dent 2012;34(3):231–8.
2. American Society of Anesthesiologists Task Force on Sedation and Analgesia by Non-Anesthesiologists. Practice guidelines for sedation and analgesia by non-anesthesiologists. Anesthesiology 2002; 96(4):1004–17.
3. American Dental Association. Guidelines for the use of sedation and general anesthesia by dentists. 2007:13.
4. Carlson ER, Sims PG. AAOMS Parameters of Care 2012. J Oral Maxillofac Surg: official journal of the American Association of Oral and Maxillofacial Surgeons 2012;70(11 Suppl 3):e1–330.
5. Stronczek MJ. Determining the appropriate oral surgery anesthesia modality, setting, and team. Oral Maxillofac Surg Clin North Am 2013;25(3):357–66, v.
6. Giovannitti JA Jr. Anesthesia for off-floor dental and oral surgery. Curr Opin Anaesthesiol 2016;29(4): 519–25.
7. Moncel JB, Nardi N, Wodey E, et al. Evaluation of the pediatric post anesthesia discharge scoring system in an ambulatory surgery unit. Paediatr Anaesth 2015;25(6):636–41.
8. Sims PG. Preoperative, intraoperative, and postoperative anesthesia assessment and monitoring in oral surgery. Oral Maxillofac Surg Clin North Am 2013;25(3):367.
9. Olkkola KT, Ahonen J. Midazolam and other benzodiazepines. Handb Exp Pharmacol 2008;(182): 335–60.
10. Pani N, Dongare PA, Mishra RK. Reversal agents in anaesthesia and critical care. Indian J Anaesth 2015;59(10):664–9.
11. Rodrigo C. Flumazenil in dentistry. Anesth Prog 1995;42(3–4):121–5.
12. Cote CJ, Karl HW, Notterman DA, et al. Adverse sedation events in pediatrics: analysis of medications used for sedation. Pediatrics 2000;106(4): 633–44.
13. Cote CJ, Notterman DA, Karl HW, et al. Adverse sedation events in pediatrics: a critical incident analysis of contributing factors. Pediatrics 2000;105(4 Pt 1):805–14.
14. Robbertze R, Posner KL, Domino KB. Closed claims review of anesthesia for procedures outside the operating room. Curr Opin Anaesthesiol 2006; 19(4):436–42.

15. Metzner J, Posner KL, Domino KB. The risk and safety of anesthesia at remote locations: the US closed claims analysis. Curr Opin Anaesthesiol 2009;22(4):502–8.

16. Gesek DJ. Respiratory anesthetic emergencies in oral and maxillofacial surgery. Oral Maxillofac Surg Clin North Am 2013;25(3):479.

17. Bennett J, Peterson T, Burleson JA. Capnography and ventilatory assessment during ambulatory dentoalveolar surgery. J Oral Maxill Surg 1997;55(9): 921–5 [discussion: 925–6].

18. Bennett JD, Kramer KJ, Bosack RC. How safe is deep sedation or general anesthesia while providing dental care? J Am Dent Assoc 2015;146(9):705–8.

19. Rosenberg H, Davis M, James D, et al. Malignant hyperthermia. Orphanet J Rare Dis 2007;2:21.

20. Sessler DI. Mild perioperative hypothermia. N Engl J Med 1997;336(24):1730–7.

21. Faust RJ, Cucchiara RF. Anesthesiology review. 3rd edition. New York: Churchill Livingstone; 2002.

22. Insler SR, Sessler DI. Perioperative thermoregulation and temperature monitoring. Anesthesiol Clin 2006; 24(4):823–37.

23. Sessler DI. Perioperative thermoregulation and heat balance. Lancet 2016;387(10038):2655–64.

24. Apfel CC, Laara E, Koivuranta M, et al. A simplified risk score for predicting postoperative nausea and vomiting: conclusions from cross-validations between two centers. Anesthesiology 1999;91(3):693–700.

25. Apfel CC, Philip BK, Cakmakkaya OS, et al. Who is at risk for postdischarge nausea and vomiting after ambulatory surgery? Anesthesiology 2012;117(3): 475–86.

26. Eberhart LH, Geldner G, Kranke P, et al. The development and validation of a risk score to predict the probability of postoperative vomiting in pediatric patients. Anesth Analg 2004;99(6):1630–7.

27. Gan TJ, Diemunsch P, Habib AS, et al. Consensus guidelines for the management of postoperative nausea and vomiting. Anesth Analg 2014;118(1): 85–113.

28. Henzi I, Walder B, Tramer MR. Dexamethasone for the prevention of postoperative nausea and vomiting: a quantitative systematic review. Anesth Analg 2000;90(1):186–94.

29. Wang JJ, Ho ST, Lee SC, et al. The use of dexamethasone for preventing postoperative nausea and vomiting in females undergoing thyroidectomy: a dose-ranging study. Anesth Analg 2000;91(6): 1404–7.

30. Wang JJ, Ho ST, Tzeng JI, et al. The effect of timing of dexamethasone administration on its efficacy as a prophylactic antiemetic for postoperative nausea and vomiting. Anesth Analg 2000;91(1):136–9.

31. Melton MS, Klein SM, Gan TJ. Management of postdischarge nausea and vomiting after ambulatory surgery. Curr Opin Anaesthesiol 2011;24(6):612–9.

32. Tramer MR, Reynolds DJ, Moore RA, et al. Efficacy, dose-response, and safety of ondansetron in prevention of postoperative nausea and vomiting: a quantitative systematic review of randomized placebo-controlled trials. Anesthesiology 1997; 87(6):1277–89.

33. Deitrick CL, Mick DJ, Lauffer V, et al. A comparison of two differing doses of promethazine for the treatment of postoperative nausea and vomiting. J Perianesth Nurs 2015;30(1):5–13.

34. Habib AS, Reuveni J, Taguchi A, et al. A comparison of ondansetron with promethazine for treating postoperative nausea and vomiting in patients who received prophylaxis with ondansetron: a retrospective database analysis. Anesth Analg 2007;104(3): 548–51.

35. Giovannitti JA, Rosenberg MB, Phero JC. Pharmacology of local anesthetics used in oral surgery. Oral Maxillofac Surg Clin North Am 2013;25(3):453.

36. Vadivelu N, Gowda AM, Urman RD, et al. Ketorolac tromethamine—routes and clinical implications. Pain Pract 2015;15(2):175–93.

37. Redden RJ. Ketorolac tromethamine: an oral/injectable nonsteroidal anti-inflammatory for postoperative pain control. J Oral Maxillofac Surg 1992; 50(12):1310–3.

38. Townsend JA, Ganzberg S, Thikkurissy S. The effect of local anesthetic on quality of recovery characteristics following dental rehabilitation under general anesthesia in children. Anesth Prog 2009;56(4): 115–22.

39. Redan JA, Wells T, Reeder S, et al. Reducing opioid adverse events: a safe way to improve outcomes. Surg Technol Int 2016;28:101–9.

40. Nishimoto RN. OFIRMEV: an old drug becomes new again. Anesth Prog 2014;61(3):99–102.

41. Badrinath S, Avramov MN, Shadrick M, et al. The use of a ketamine-propofol combination during monitored anesthesia care. Anesth Analg 2000; 90(4):858–62.

42. Slavik VC, Zed PJ. Combination ketamine and propofol for procedural sedation and analgesia. Pharmacotherapy 2007;27(11):1588–98.

43. Bell RF, Dahl JB, Moore RA, et al. Peri-operative ketamine for acute post-operative pain: a quantitative and qualitative systematic review (Cochrane review). Acta Anaesthesiol Scand 2005;49(10):1405–28.

44. Agarwal R, Porter MH, Obeid G. Common medical illnesses that affect anesthesia and their anesthetic management. Oral Maxillofac Surg Clin North Am 2013;25(3):407.

45. Vasu TS, Grewal R, Doghramji K. Obstructive sleep apnea syndrome and perioperative complications: a systematic review of the literature. J Clin Sleep Med 2012;8(2):199–207.

46. Finkel KJ, Searleman AC, Tymkew H, et al. Prevalence of undiagnosed obstructive sleep apnea

among adult surgical patients in an academic medical center. Sleep Med 2009;10(7):753–8.

47. Vasu TS, Doghramji K, Cavallazzi R, et al. Obstructive sleep apnea syndrome and postoperative complications: clinical use of the STOP-BANG questionnaire. Arch Otolaryngol Head Neck Surg 2010;136(10):1020–4.

48. American Society of Anesthesiologists Task Force on Perioperative Management of patients with obstructive sleep apnea. Practice guidelines for the perioperative management of patients with obstructive sleep apnea: an updated report by the American Society of Anesthesiologists Task Force on Perioperative Management of patients with obstructive sleep apnea. Anesthesiology 2014;120(2):268–86.

49. Huang A, Tanbonliong T. Oral sedation postdischarge adverse events in pediatric dental patients. Anesth Prog 2015;62(3):91–9.

50. Todd DW. Pediatric sedation and anesthesia for the oral surgeon. Oral Maxillofac Surg Clin North Am 2013;25(3):467.

51. Martinez D, Wilson S. Children sedated for dental care: a pilot study of the 24-hour postsedation period. Pediatr Dent 2006;28(3):260–4.

Equipment Safety, Maintenance and Inspection
What the Oral Surgeon Needs to Know

Katherine A. Keeley, DDS, MD

KEYWORDS

- Equipment maintenance • Patient safety • Office-based surgery • Biomedical testing
- Equipment calibration • Sterilization monitoring • Radiation safety and monitoring
- Nitrous oxide sedation

KEY POINTS

- Equipment requires annual biomedical testing and calibration.
- Process indicators, spore tests, and regular maintenance assure sterilizer effectiveness.
- Radiation survey can be satisfied by short-term dosimetry badge wearing or an area monitor.
- Medical gases need to be properly stored and monitored to decrease risks to patients and staff.
- Back-up power and lighting are needed for critical equipment during an electrical failure.

INTRODUCTION

Many oral and maxillofacial surgical procedures are done in an office-based setting, with many oral and maxillofacial surgeons (OMSs) directly or indirectly involved in oversight of equipment maintenance. Goals in equipment management are to prevent harm to patients and staff, stay compliant with current regulations, and increase equipment longevity where possible. Harm to patients or staff can happen when there is electrical leak from equipment, inaccurate vital sign data, an improperly functioning autoclave, excessive radiation, incorrect plumbing of anesthetic gases, or loss of light and/or power during a procedure or resuscitative event. Fortunately, the steps needed to prevent equipment-related mishaps are straightforward and easy to implement.[1,2] There are few data on equipment-related events in office-based surgery, but in a review of sentinel events reported to the Joint Commission (JC) in 2012, medical equipment-related incidents were only the tenth most common type of incident. Of those incidents, greater than 82% of them were caused by human factors, not mechanical failure. Even if the number of cases may be small, the consequences can be catastrophic, as in the case of errors in the administration and storage of medical gases. It is imperative to always follow the manufacturer's recommendations and train all employees in the proper use and maintenance of all medical equipment.

Regulatory compliance is becoming more of a concern for the office-based OMS, especially those that are medically licensed. In the past, the sometimes voluntary, state-run, Office Anesthesia Evaluation (OAE) program[3] was the only regularly recurring inspection an OMS would face, every 5 years. The OAE is required to maintain American Association of Oral and Maxillofacial Surgeons (AAOMS) membership[4] and assesses an office for appropriate anesthesia rescue equipment and drugs as well as tests the provider on his or her knowledge of the management of medical emergencies. The inspection checks for presence of

Private Practice, 2649 Wigwam Parkway, Suite #102, Henderson, NV 89074, USA
E-mail address: kakeeleyomfs@yahoo.com

Oral Maxillofacial Surg Clin N Am 29 (2017) 209–221
http://dx.doi.org/10.1016/j.coms.2016.12.012
1042-3699/17/© 2017 Elsevier Inc. All rights reserved.

equipment, but not functionality of equipment, or current inspection and certification of equipment. In many states, as an MD licensed OMS, one would not even be subjected to the OAE for an anesthesia permit since many states did not, and at least 25 still do not, require certification for an MD to do office-based anesthesia or surgery.[5,6] As more surgical procedures go to the outpatient setting, and surgical and anesthetic mishaps in the office setting continue to be high profile, there has been a push for more regulation.[7] The regulations, when enacted by state legislatures, apply to MD licensed OMSs, and stem from Centers for Medicare and Medicaid Services (CMS) conditions of participation that apply to inpatient facilities. CMS relies on accrediting organizations (OAs) to survey facilities with state agencies conducting audits or validation surveys. This is the same model usually utilized for affected MD office-based anesthesia offices. The 3 national organizations that offer accreditation of office-based surgical facilities are the American Association for the Accreditation of Ambulatory Surgical Facilities (AAAASF), Association for the Accreditation of Ambulatory Healthcare (AAAHC), and the JC (**Box 1**). Most states also do a yearly site visit. The tests and procedures for optimal equipment safety and maintenance discussed in this article are those usually required by these governing agencies and the relevant state and federal organizations.

This article will cover the safety, maintenance, and inspection related to electrical equipment used in the treatment of patients, autoclaves, radiograph machines, nitrous oxide and oxygen medical gases, and required back-up power and lighting. In all cases the office should follow manufacturer's recommendations regarding maintenance and inspection, and document policies and monitoring so compliance can be proved to governing bodies.

ELECTRICAL SAFETY AND CALIBRATION

All medical/surgical equipment needs to be on a program of scheduled preventive maintenance and calibration, done by a credible biomedical service vendor.[8] All electrical equipment in the patient treatment areas, and other major medical electric equipment like a sterilizer or radiology machine, must be tested (**Table 1**). Electrical safety inspection helps prevent the hazards of using defective or improperly grounded electric medical equipment. The biomedical service provider will inventory equipment by manufacturer, type, model, and serial number. This should be done annually and a log book kept with the inspection reports (**Table 2**). Anesthesia machines should be tested from 1 to 4 times a year, depending on the manufacturer and type of machine. After the equipment is tested, a sticker is placed on the item with the date and year of the inspection and when it expires (**Fig. 1**).

The inspection is a test to ensure that equipment is working within the acceptable safety parameters set out by the National Fire Protection Association (NFPA) and the Association for Advancement of Medical Instrumentation (AAMI). Both organizations are nonprofit organizations devoted to reducing hazards in health care through the development of standards, research, training, and education. When these voluntary standards are adopted by CMS or other government agencies in their licensing requirements, like NFPA's Standards for Health Care Facilities,[9] they become mandatory requirements for hospitals, and as an extension, the outpatient Accrediting Organizations (AO)s.[10]

Box 1
National accrediting bodies for office-based anesthesia practices

Accreditation Association for Ambulatory Health Care (AAAHC)
5250 Old Orchard Road, Suite 200
Skokie, IL 60077
www.aaahc.org

American Association for Accreditation of Ambulatory Surgery Facilities (AAAASF)
5101 Washington Street, Suite 2F
Gurnee, IL 60031
www.aaaasf.org

The Joint Commission (JC)
One Renaissance Boulevard
Oakbrook Terrace, IL 60181
www.jointcommission.org

Table 1
Equipment requiring electrical testing and calibration

Patient Treatment Room Equipment	Major Medical Electrical Equipment
Vital signs monitors	Sterilizer
Electric drill consoles	Radiology equipment
Headlight	
X-Ray viewer	
Dental/surgical chair	
Portable suction unit	
Automated external defibrillator/ Defibrillators	
Anesthesia machine[a]	

[a] Electrical testing and calibration should be done from 1 to 4 times per year, depending on the manufacturer.

Table 2
Sample equipment inventory safety form

Equip ID	Type	MFT	Model	Serial	M Ohms	Norm Leakage	Worse Case Leakage	Polarity	Amps	Comments
13,200	EKG/BP OX	Criticare	8100EP	407031428	148	0.20	47.00	ORP	0.10	Calibrated
14,569	Chair Lamp	Belmont	Bel-20	061317399	167	0.1	71.00	ORP	4.40	Lamp rewired
14,554	AED	Burdick	9200RD-001	320496	—	—	—	Inspected	—	Pads and battery OK

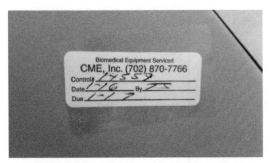

Fig. 1. Biomedical service provider sticker on a piece of equipment.

All components of a vital sign monitor including the electrocardiogram (ECG), pulse-oximetry, noninvasive blood pressure, and temperature are calibrated by the biomedical service provider. Carbon dioxide calibration is recommended to be done yearly by most manufacturers, but is not required by regulation. If one resides in a state requiring survey and accreditation for an MD licensed provider, one will likely be surveyed by both the state and AO for compliance with electrical testing and calibration.

In general, these regulations are not enforced by the Office Anesthesia Evaluation or dental boards. It is suggested in the OAE Guidelines that monitoring equipment should be checked and calibrated in accordance with manufacturer's recommendations, but it is not part of the OAE Evaluation Form, and electrical testing of other equipment is not mentioned (**Table 3**).[3] Equipment calibration and electrical testing should be added to the OAE. This is an easy way to increase patient safety and bring all OMS offices to a higher standard in line with other specialties performing outpatient surgery and anesthesia.

Sterilizer Maintenance for Patient Safety and Equipment Longevity

Rules regarding infection control and maintenance of one's sterilizer come through the Centers for Disease Control and Prevention (CDC), and are enforced through state boards of health and frequently the state dental board.[11] Regardless of the state and one's licensure status, surveillance regarding these standards is likely, and is absolutely essential to ensure one is not transmitting disease between patients. Logs will need to be kept regarding the tests run on sterilizer loads to show the contents are adequately sterilized and on the regular maintenance of the sterilizer, assuring proper functioning.

Due to speed of processing, safety, and cost, the most common sterilizer used for the heat-tolerant instruments used in OMS practices is a steam sterilizer, or autoclave. Other high-heat sterilizers

include dry heat and unsaturated chemical vapor. Low-heat sterilizers take more time and are more commonly used in large facilities (**Table 4**).

The CDC requires all instruments to be placed in a pouch or wrapped in a way to allow penetration of the sterilization agent and storage of the instruments to keep them sterile until used.[11] An unwrapped cycle, or flash sterilization, should only be used for instruments that will be used immediately. To assure successful sterilization, several process indicators, specific for the type of sterilizer, are used. Maintain a log that records spore test and integrator results on every autoclave run (**Table 5**). This allows one to reference and evaluate the load if ever an indicator or spore test were to fail.

Type 1, or external process indicators, are used on the outside of every pouch or wrapped cassette to essentially show whether or not it has been processed. In addition, an internal process indicator is needed inside every pouch or wrapped cassette to show whether the contents of the package were adequately sterilized (**Table 6**).

Many of the pouches purchased for sterilization have both an external (Type I) and internal process indicator (Type IV) built in (**Fig. 2**). A color change in one or both after a sterilizer run shows that certain minimum standards of the sterilization process have been met (ie, the correct temperature and pressure for the appropriate period of time) (**Figs. 3** and **4**).

In addition, the more sensitive biologic spore test (BI) monitoring, with a control as well, must be done weekly, at a minimum, and recorded. Unlike mechanical and chemical indicators that evaluate conditions of sterilization, the biologic spore test is an evaluation of sterilizer effectiveness. The spore test evaluates killing of highly resistant spores and in higher numbers than would ever be seen in one's sterilizer load.

If an indicator fails to change color or you fail a spore test, it indicates either something is wrong with the sterilizer or the load was packed incorrectly. Check the sterilizer maintenance log and load contents. One will want to send another test and investigate as soon as possible.[12]

Frequently offices utilize mail-in sterilization monitoring services with a 2- to 3-day delay. This delay can be overcome by doing one's own on-site spore testing or by incorporating the use of a Type V integrating indicator in each autoclave run (see **Table 6**).

Type V is the most accurate internal chemical indicator and reacts to values that are equivalent to or exceed that of a BI, or spore test. The Type V integrator provides immediate results so one can release processed instruments with confidence.

Table 3
Regulatory framework for equipment-related safety issues

	Electrical Safety and Calibration	Autoclave Sterilization and Maintenance	Radiation Safety	Medical Gases	Back-up Power, Light and Suction
Enforced by OAE	No[a]	No	No	Yes	Yes
Enforced by accrediting organizations	Yes	Yes	Yes	Yes	Yes
City or state enforcing agency	State agency within board of health or quality for those MD licensed in affected states	State Board of health and dental boards	State or federal OSHA program and state radiation control division	City/county fire safety; state or federal OSHA program	
Nonprofit organization guiding legislation	National Fire Protection Association and Association for the Advancement of Medical Instrumentation (AAMI)		Conference of Radiation Control Program Directors	National Fire Protection Association	
Federal Agency	CMS	CDC	OSHA	OSHA, CDC	
US department	Department of Health and Human Services (DHSS)	Department of Health and Human Services (DHSS)	Department of Labor	Department Of Labor, DHSS	

[a] Suggested in Evaluation Guidelines that equipment should be checked and calibrated in accordance with manufacturer's recommendations, but it is not part of the evaluation form.

Table 4
Types of sterilizers

Sterilizer	Advantages	Disadvantages
Types of high heat sterilizers		
Steam under pressure (autoclave)	Short processing times, low cost, reliable, low risk to staff	Can be corrosive to some instruments because of moisture
Dry heat	Noncorrosive; low cost	Longer processing times; high temperaturs can be damaging
Chemical vapor (solution of primarily alcohol mixed with 0.23% formaldehyde)	Less corrosive than steam on carbon steel instruments	Safety and regulation issues due to hazardous waste; instruments must be dry before sterilizing
Types of low heat sterilizers		
Ethylene oxide gas (ETO)	Sterilize heat and moisture sensitive items; easy to operate (used in larger health care facilities)	Long sterilization times of 10–48 h; stringent health and safety requirements due to toxicity; not useful for handpieces
Hydrogen peroxide gas plasma	Sterilize heat and moisture sensitive items; safe for environment; no toxic residuals (used in larger healthcare facilities)	Not effective for some instruments with long or narrow lumens; requires synthetic packaging

From Rutala WA. Guidelines for disinfection and sterilization in healthcare facilities. Atlanta (GA): CDC; 2008. p. 110–1.

When performing a spore test, it is important to place the testing strip in the most challenging area of the autoclave and place it in the most representative load on the day testing is done. This is usually the most anterior aspect of the central tray and within a pouch or wrapped cassette.

To assure appropriate functioning and long-term viability of the autoclave it is important to perform daily, weekly, and monthly maintenance and record it in a log (**Table 7**). Always refer to the manufacturer's recommendations for specifics. Only use distilled water in a steam sterilizer

Table 5
Sample steam sterilization log

Sterilizer	Date	Load #	Time	Operator Initials	Load Contents	Parameters/ Cycle	Quality Control	Results	
M11 Statim 2000					TR1 FOR BB SRK ME IDK BOW DR MG SYR	Pouch Wrapped Unwrapped	Spore test? Result Chem Indic Change	Yes Pass Yes	No Fail No
M11 Statim 2000					TR1 FOR BB SRK ME IDK BOW DR MG SYR	Pouch Wrapped Unwrapped	Spore test? Result Chem Indic Change	Yes Pass Yes	No Fail No
M11 Statim 2000					TR1 FOR BB SRK ME IDK BOW DR IA SYR	Pouch Wrapped Unwrapped	Spore test? Result Chem Indic Change	Yes Pass Yes	No Fail No

Abbreviations: BB, bite block; BOW, bowls; DR, drill; FOR, forceps; IDK, Implant drill kit; ME, mirror, explorer; MG, mouth gags; SRK, suture removal kit; SYR, syringe, etc; TR1, tray 1 set-up of instruments.

Table 6
Steam chemical indicator types

Steam Chemical Indicator Types[a]	Definition
Type I Process Indicators	For use on the exterior of individual packs to show exposure to the sterilization process.
Type II Indicators for use in specific tests	For use in specific test procedures (eg, the Bowie-Dick Test that evaluates steam penetration)
Type III Single variable indicators	Indicates exposure to a single critical variable of the sterilization process (eg, a temperature tube with a chemical pellet that melts at a certain temperature)
Type IV Multivariable indicators	An internal indicator used inside a pack that reacts to two or more of the critical variables of the sterilization process (only available for steam sterilizers)
Type V Integrating indicators	The most accurate of the internal chemical indicators; reacts to all critical variables of the sterilization process, and the stated values are equivalent to or exceed BI performance requirements; gives immediate definitive results
Type VI Emulating indicators	An internal chemical indicator that reacts to all critical variables of the sterilization process for a specified sterilization cycle

[a] There is no significance to the rank order of the type of indicator.
From American National Standards Institute/Association for the Advancement of Medical Instrumentation/International Organization for Standardization. Sterilization of health care products – chemical indicators – part 1: general requirements. Arlington (VA): AAMI; 2014. p. 11140–1.

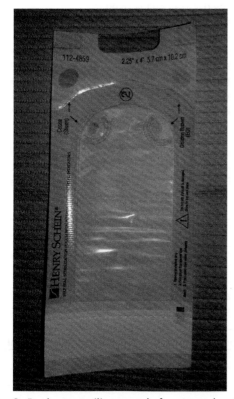

and for cleaning. At high temperatures, any dissolved minerals or particles in tap water will deposit on the metal surfaces causing build-up and corrosion, which will interfere with function over time. When cleaning the external or internal components of the sterilizer, only use quaternary ammonia compounds due to their noncorrosive properties. A log book of the cleaning schedule for the autoclave(s) is essential since inconsistent maintenance is a cause for inadequate sterilization and breakdown of the machine.

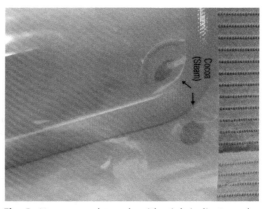

Fig. 2. Dual use sterilizer pouch for steam (on the *left* and *pink*) and ethylene oxide (on the *right* and *blue*). (Henry Schein, Melville, NY)

Fig. 3. Unprocessed pouch with pink indicator color for both the internal process indicator (*left*) and external process indicator (*right*).

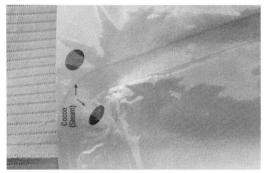

Fig. 4. Processed pouch with cocoa indicator color for both the internal process indicator (*left*) and external process indicator (*right*).

RADIATION SAFETY IN RELATION TO DIAGNOSTIC RADIATION EQUIPMENT

Regulations pertaining to radiation safety come from the Radiation Control Division of the Occupational Safety and Health Administration (OSHA), an agency of the US Department of Labor.[13] The regulations adopted by state legislators and state radiation protection programs are essentially those recommended by the Conference of Radiation Control Program Directors, Incorporated (CRCPD). This nonprofit organization is made up of the radiation control programs of 50 states, District of Columbia, and Puerto Rico. Their mission is to review current data and regulations, develop task forces as needed, and to come out with recommendations on regulations that will help protect the public, radiation workers, and patients from unnecessary radiation exposure.[14] They develop regulations that are usually adopted by all the states.

The first rule in radiation safety is to make every effort to keep the exposure to radiation as low as is reasonably achievable, or the ALARA (As Low As Reasonably Achievable) principle, in conducting radiographic exams.[15] Radiation protection programs vary by state, but in general require one to register new radiologic equipment and renew registration yearly. This will be followed by an initial inspection of the equipment and office looking at general operation and safety. Next, a radiation survey is required to assess radiation hazards present in the operation of the machine in the location it is placed.[10,16] This can be done by a medical physicist or area monitor. The medical physicist calculates expected radiation by looking at geometry and workload. If the area monitor or personnel dosimetry badges worn for 3 months receive less than 10% of the maximum allowed dose of radiation per year (**Table 8**),[13] then one can stop monitoring unless something changes with a new machine or change in geometry of the area where films are taken. Send survey information to the state's Radiation Control Division and ask for written verification that the radiation survey requirements have been satisfied. Maintain this in your records to document compliance.[17] With the advent of digital radiography, radiation exposure to staff is frequently negligible, and further monitoring is not necessary (**Table 9**). Continuous badge wearing of personnel whole body and extremity dose monitoring devices is required if a handheld X-Ray unit is used.[18]

The AOs require the monitoring devices or processes necessary to ensure safety of all personnel who might be exposed to radiation, but not continuous monitoring.[19] Records of this compliance along with radiation exposure reports of all employees must be kept. In reviewing OSHA standards, a log book of any dosimetry badge reports should be kept for the lifetime of the employee and practice. All offices can expect to be surveyed on these radiation standards by state or federal OSHA programs or state Radiation Control Divisions. If one is accredited, surveillance on

Table 7
Sample steam sterilizer maintenance log

Week of the Year	Date	Drain and Replace Distilled Water Weekly	Clean Chamber and Trays Weekly	Flush System × 3 Incl. with Cleaner in Chamber Monthly	Clean Chamber Filters Monthly	Perform Pressure Valve Relief Check Monthly	Remove and Clean Door Gasket Monthly	Initials
1								
2								
3								

Maintenance should always be performed according to manufacturer's recommendations. Daily maintenance includes checking the distilled water level, cleaning external surfaces, and cleaning and checking the door gasket.

Table 8
Dose limits of ionizing radiation

	Rems[a] per Calendar Quarter
Whole body: head and trunk, active blood-forming organs, lens of eyes, or gonads	1.25
Hands and forearms; feet and ankles	18.75
Skin of whole body	7.5

[a] Rem is a measure of the dose of any ionizing radiation to body tissue in terms of its estimated biological effect relative to a dose of 1 R (r) of radiographs (1 mrem (mrem) = 0.001 rem).

these requirements will still be required, except the length of time required to keep employee exposure data may be less.

Pregnant employees can continue to work with diagnostic radiology equipment. However, one should evaluate their work environment and make adjustments as necessary to be sure they have a low risk of receiving a radiation dose. These employees may request dosimetry badge monitoring while they are pregnant, and one may decide to alter their job description to limit possible radiation exposure as much as possible.[20]

MEDICAL GASES

Mixtures of nitrous oxide (N_2O) and oxygen (O_2) have been used as analgesic and sedative agents in dentistry and OMS for over 100 years. The usual equipment includes central tank storage and an N_2O and O_2 delivery system, a gas mixing bag, and a nasal mask with a positive pressure relief valve. Several regulatory agencies are involved due to the risks to patients and staff, and facility risks due to storage and plumbing of the gases.

During N_2O sedation, the greatest risk to the patient is oxygen deprivation, which can lead to death. These rare, catastrophic events can happen from incorrect initial plumbing of the lines or other line mix-ups or failures down the road that result in a gas mixture to the patient with less than 20% oxygen.[21] All newly installed OMS facilities that have piped medical gases or deliver N_2O must be checked by city plumbing and fire safety inspectors for proper gas delivery and fail-safe function prior to use (**Fig. 5**).[9] The inhalation equipment must have the capacity for delivering 100% O_2, and the fail-safe mechanism prevents a N_2O mixture of less than 30% O_2. If the O_2 tanks are stored remotely, at least 2 tanks of O_2 must be connected to the system so the second tank can be activated if the line pressure drops in the first. If an automatic changeover system is used, an audible or visual alarm is required to notify that reserves are being used.[3] The Pin Indexing Safety System (PISS) uses unique geometry for the placement of pins on the yokes, or connectors, of each type of gas (**Figs. 6** and **7**). This helps prevent the incorrect connection of a yoke to a machine using pressurized gases. Despite these

Table 9
Sample and typical radiation exposure report

Employee Name and Identifiers	Badge Type	Body Region	Monitoring Period		Current Exposure		Quarter to Date		Year to Date		Lifetime to Date	
Last, first ID#	TLD[a] 760 Badge	WB[b]	1st day of Qtr	Last day of Qtr	Deep Eye Shallow Neutron	* * * *	Deep Eye Shallow Neutron	0 0 0 0	Deep Eye Shallow Neutron	0 0 0 0	Deep Eye Shallow Neutron	0 0 0 0
Last, first ID#	TLD[a] 760 Badge	WB[b]	1st day of Qtr	Last day of Qtr	Deep Eye Shallow Neutron	* * * *	Deep Eye Shallow Neutron	0 0 0 0	Deep Eye Shallow Neutron	0 0 0 0	Deep Eye Shallow Neutron	0 0 0 0

Dose equivalent in millirems (1 mrem = 0.001 rem) for time periods indicated.
[a] Thermoluminescent dosimeter responding to neutron, gamma, beta, and X-radiation.
[b] Whole body.
* Undetectable level.

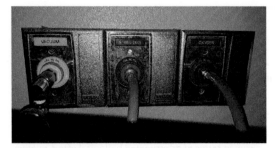

Fig. 5. Typical office set up with a vacuum line, N_2O and O_2.

measures, the safest way to prevent hypoxia is to also have a qualitative O_2 sensor in the line delivering N_2O/O_2 gas to the patient.[21]

Long-term exposure or chronic abuse of N_2O can have catastrophic effects due to its interference with methionine synthetase and resultant decreased B12 levels. This can lead to bone marrow suppression, immunologic and reproductive disturbances, neuropathy, and irreversible myeloneuropathy.[22] Excessive exposure to N_2O can occur from leaks in the anesthetic delivery system at multiple points from the tanks to the patient. Inspect and maintain all hoses, connectors, and fittings and repair leaks immediately. An appropriate scavenging system must be present.[3,23] This is usually accomplished by a vacuum line attached to the nasal mask, with a one-way valve, venting the patient's exhaled gases to the outside at a steady flow rate of 45 L/min, measured by a calibrated flow device (**Fig. 8**). To help prevent adverse health effects from N_2O, assure appropriate room ventilation with 100% clean outdoor air for the operatory and utilize an additional exhaust hood near the patient's mouth.

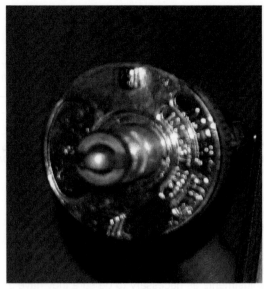

Fig. 7. PISS with N_2O pins set at 185° to each other.

NIOSH (The National Institute for Occupational Safety and Health) also recommends periodic sampling of N_2O levels in the personal breathing zone. This can be done real time with a portable infrared gas analyzer or with a personnel worn dosimetry badge that is exposed during a patient anesthetic.[24] It is then sent to an outside laboratory for analysis. This allows one to identify high N_2O levels and act accordingly to identify and fix problems.

Cylinders containing O_2 and N_2O gas are under high pressure and can be a combustion, explosion, fire, and projectile hazard. If O_2 has exposure to hydrocarbons like oil or grease, there is also a significant combustion hazard. Because of this, OSHA and NFPA standards require oxygen cylinders be stored in a well-protected, ventilated

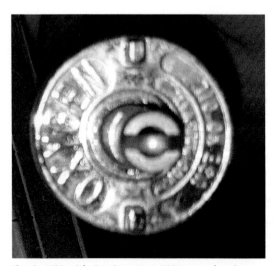

Fig. 6. PISS with O_2 pins set at 180° to each other.

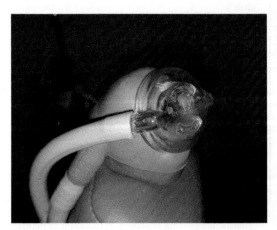

Fig. 8. N2O/O2 nasal mask. One of the tubes is attached to the vacuum line to remove exhaled gases.

area and secured so they cannot be knocked over (**Fig. 9**). Appropriate signage needs to be at all facility entrances (**Fig. 10**) and on the doors where the cylinders are located (**Fig. 11**).

In addition to an initial office inspection, all OMS offices are required by local regulators to have a yearly fire safety inspection where appropriate storage of the tanks and room ventilation will be evaluated. This will also be evaluated by the OAE and AOs. The OAE will assess whether fail-safe flow meters and alarms are in place to protect patients from hypoxic events and that measures are in place to control N_2O exposure. AOs may further evaluate that the practice is monitoring the levels of N_2O gas in the environment.[25]

BACK-UP POWER AND LIGHTING

Some source of emergency power (battery or generator) is needed to power any critical equipment in order to complete a procedure or resuscitation during an electrical failure. For oral and maxillofacial surgery, this requires an auxiliary form of light and suction to complete the procedure at hand as well as auxiliary oxygen and a battery backed-up vital sign monitor in case the patient is under anesthesia. The lighting system should be mobile and can be a battery powered flashlight or headlight (**Fig. 12**). The portable suction unit can have a constantly charging back-up battery (**Fig. 13**), and the portable oxygen unit needs to be capable of delivering oxygen under positive pressure for at least an hour (**Fig. 14**).[23] Frequently, there is a green light illuminated on the front of the vital signs monitor to show the battery is functional (**Fig. 15**). It turns red when the battery needs to be changed. Offices will be inspected for these items by the OAE and AOs.

It is recommended to do a monthly safety check of proper battery function of back-up equipment and record it in a log.[26] One may find it more convenient to check battery function of backup equipment at the same time one is doing weekly

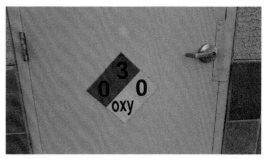

Fig. 10. Sign placed at all entry points to the facility.

checks of the AED battery and other resuscitative equipment. In addition, some AOs require the batteries for the building emergency lighting to be replaced annually, even though the life of the battery may be longer. If there is a generator for back-up power, at least monthly it needs to be tested under load for 30 continuous minutes.[25]

SUMMARY/DISCUSSION

In the last 10 years, there has been an increase in the number of regulations with which an OMS needs to be in compliance. This is especially seen in the states requiring accreditation of office-based practices administering general anesthesia. Although many regulations are costly and time-consuming, there are benefits in improving office safety and efficiency and preventing patient harm. Fortunately, complying with recommendations on equipment safety and maintenance is straightforward, inexpensive, and easy.

For electrical testing and calibration, the process can be referred out to a biomedical service provider who also provides a written report to show

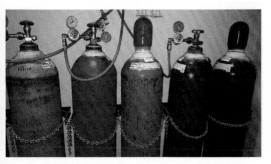

Fig. 9. Medical gas tanks stored with chains to prevent tipping.

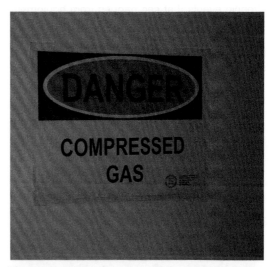

Fig. 11. Sign placed on door of the medical gas storage area.

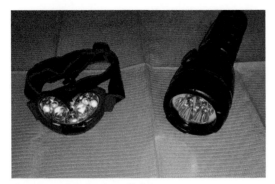

Fig. 12. Mobile back-up lighting.

compliance. Keep appropriate logs on sterilizer maintenance, runs, and spore tests, and use personnel dosimetry badges or area monitors long enough to establish safe levels of radiation exposure. Work with the local fire department during initial set-up of the office and complete an inspection before any medical gases are administered. To further prevent harm, utilize an oxygen sensor in the gas line to the patient. Use appropriate scavenging systems to limit staff exposure to N_2O and properly store all medical gases. Appropriate back-up power and lighting help prevent untoward events in the event of a power failure. In all cases, follow manufacturer recommendations and refer to your state for specifics on regulations. Written policies and documentation of compliance are essential to stay on track and present to regulators.

I have always felt regulations should be evaluated for their benefit to patients and society, while keeping in mind their cost to implement. Compliance with the equipment safety and maintenance recommendations in this article is an easy way to prevent a small number of potentially catastrophic events that can happen from equipment malfunction.

However, there is currently wide variation in the regulations followed by OMS offices related to the state one resides in and licensure status, and

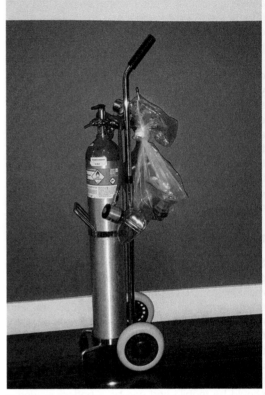

Fig. 14. Portable O_2 with positive pressure delivery capability.

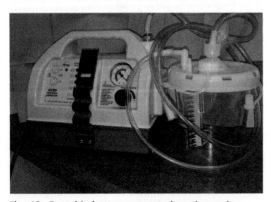

Fig. 13. Portable battery-operated suction unit.

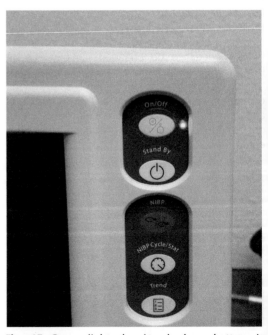

Fig. 15. Green light showing back-up battery is functional.

whether or not that requires one to be accredited. The nonaccredited office is subjected to far fewer regulations and inspections. As expectations for quality of care in office-based surgery continue to increase, the time has come to elevate standards and have them apply to all, regardless of accreditation requirements. This will benefit patients and our specialty, and allow doctors to maintain the privilege of offering outpatient surgery and anesthesia in their offices.

REFERENCES

1. The Joint Commission. Medical device alarm safety in hospitals. Sentinel Event Alert 2013;(50):1–3.
2. Perrott D. Outcomes of clinical practice of oral and maxillofacial surgery. J Oral Maxillofac Surg 2003; 61:983–95.
3. American Association of Oral and Maxillofacial Surgeons. Office anesthesia evaluation manual. 8th edition. Rosemont (IL): AAOMS; 2012.
4. American Association of Oral and Maxillofacial Surgeons. Governing rules and regulations. Chapter III, Section 30. Rosemont (IL): AAOMS; 2016–2017.
5. Federation of State Medical Boards. State Board requirements for office-based surgery A-M. Available at: https://www.fsmb.org/Media/Default/PDF/FSMB/Advocacy/GRPOL_Office_Based_Surgery_A-M.pdf. Accessed October 30, 2016.
6. Federation of State Medical Boards. State Board requirements for office-based surgery N-Z. Available at: https://www.fsmb.org/Media/Default/PDF/FSMB/Advocacy/GRPOL_Office_Based_Surgery_N-Z.pdf. Accessed October 30, 2016.
7. Todd D, Nannini V, Kelling T, et al. Office accreditation experiences with 3 accrediting agencies and suggestions for changes in private oral and maxillofacial surgery facility evaluations. J Oral Maxillofac Surg 2011;69:258–70.
8. Core Chapter 8, N: Facilities and EnvironmentAccreditation handbook for office-based surgery including review guidelines. AAAHC; 2016.
9. National Fire Protection Association. NFPA – 99: health care facilities code. Quincy (MA): NFPA; 2015. Sec 5.1.3.2.1–14.
10. Wang B. Medical equipment maintenance: management and oversight. San Rafael (CA): Morgan and Claypool; 2012.
11. Centers for Disease Control and Prevention. Guidelines for infection control in dental health care settings. MMWR 2003;52:22–5.
12. Rutala WA. Guidelines for disinfection and sterilization in healthcare facilities. Atlanta (GA): CDC; 2008.
13. Occupational Safety and Health Administration. Occupational safety and health standards: ionizing radiation – 1910.1096. Standards – 29 CFR. OSHA; 1996. p. 1–13 (09-2015), (a-p).
14. The Conference of Radiation Control Program Directors. CRCPD: the continuing saga 1993-2007. Available at: http://www.crcpd.org/Pubs/CRCPD-TheContinuingSaga.pdf.
15. Nevada Administrative Code NAC 459.0205 "As low as is reasonably achievable" defined. Available at: http://www.leg.state.nv.us/nac/nac-459.html#NAC459Sec0205.
16. Nevada Administrative Code NAC 459.337 surveys and monitoring. Available at: http://www.leg.state.nv.us/nac/nac-459.html#NAC459Sec337.
17. Nevada Administrative Code NAC 459.3645 NAC 459.3645 records of surveys and calibrations. Available at: http://www.leg.state.nv.us/nac/nac-459.html#NAC459Sec3645.
18. Nevada Administrative Code NAC 459.5595 requirements for registrants of portable equipment which is hand-held and facilities which house such equipment. Available at: http://www.leg.state.nv.us/nac/nac-459.html#NAC459Sec5595.
19. Accreditation handbook for office-based surgery including review guidelines. Adjunct Chapter 13: Diagnostic and other Imaging Services. AAAHC; 2016. p. 82.
20. International Commission on Radiologic Protection. Pregnancy and medical radiation. ICRP Publication 84. Ann ICRP 2000;30(1). Available at: http://www.icrp.org/publication.asp?id=ICRP%20Publication%2084.
21. Goho C, Kittle P. Override of an N2O/O2 machine fail-safe mechanism: Case report. Pediatr Dent 1991;13(4):234–5.
22. Stacey CB, Di Rocco A, Gould RJ. Methionine in the treatment of nitrous-oxide induced neuropathy and myeloneuropathy. J Neurol 1992;7:401–3.
23. American Association of Oral and Maxillofacial Surgeons. Parameters of care: clinical practice guidelines for oral and maxillofacial surgery. Anesthesia in outpatient facilities. Rosemont (IL): AAOMS; 2012.
24. National Institute for Occupational Safety and Health. NIOSH hazard control—control of nitrous oxide in dental operatories 1998; DHHS (NIOSH) Publication No. 96-107. Available at: http://www.cdc.gov/niosh/docs/hazardcontrol/hc3.html.
25. The Joint Commission. Comprehensive accreditation manual for office-based surgery practices. Oak Brook (IL): JC; 2015.
26. American Association for Accreditation of Ambulatory Surgery Facilities, Inc. Oral and Maxillofacial Surgery Facility Standards and Checklist 2011, Version 2. p. 40.

Patient Safety and the Malpractice System

James Q. Swift, DDS

KEYWORDS

• Tort system • Risk management • Informed consent • Patient safety

KEY POINTS

- The cost of health care in the United States and malpractice insurance has escalated greatly over the past 30 years.
- In an ideal world, the goals of the tort system would be aligned with efforts at improving safety.
- There is little evidence that the tort system and the processes of risk management and informed consent have improved patient safety.

The cost of health care in the United States has increased dramatically over the past few decades. There are many explanations offered as to why this has occurred, including the use and implementation of newly designed and costly devices and implants; the introduction of novel pharmaceutical agents that are expensive to develop, test, and bring to market; and the costs of health care education and health care delivery infrastructure.

One frequent cited and significant contributing factor is the cost associated with the malpractice epidemic, which has developed, persisted, and escalated largely over the past 30 years. Although malpractice insurance premiums across the board have stabilized in the past decade, and frequency and severity of claims have leveled, the cost of the entire enterprise is stifling. According to Hilary Clinton and Barack Obama, "high premiums are forcing physicians to give up performing certain high risk procedures leaving patients without access to a full range of medical services."[1] They also claim that "the tort system must achieve four goals: reduce the rates of preventable patient injuries, promote open communication between physicians and patient, ensure patients access to fair compensation for legitimate medical injuries and reduce liability insurance premiums for health care providers."[1]

There is little, if any, objective evidence that the tort system has even scratched the surface in achieving these lofty and largely unachievable objectives. The cost of defensive medicine also adds to the cost. Examples include prescribing antibiotics when not indicated to supplant the risk of an unlikely occurrence of a serious infection, exposing patients to the cost and risk of loss of bacterial susceptibility to a therapeutic medication. Another example is exposure of a patient to a preoperative cone beam CT scan for fear that if a complication occurs, an expert witness may allege that the standard of care was violated when that study was not ordered. Several examples occur in medicine. One is the recommended frequency of mammograms for evaluation for potential breast cancer. If a national agency or body determines that the frequency between mammograms be expanded as a general rule, a patient who experiences breast cancer within the extended interval may feel that the frequency of evaluation should have been greater. And if an expert can be located who agrees, a lawsuit may be filed.

The tort system has been labeled adversarial, promoting a behavior of defensiveness, denial, and blame. The concept of error disclosure has been aligned by some people with the patient

Advanced Specialty Education in Oral and Maxillofacial Surgery, Division of Oral and Maxillofacial Surgery, University of Minnesota, 7-174 Moos Tower, School of Dentistry, 515 Delaware St. SE, Minneapolis, MN 55455 0329, USA

E-mail address: Swift001@umn.edu

Oral Maxillofacial Surg Clin N Am 29 (2017) 223–227
http://dx.doi.org/10.1016/j.coms.2016.12.010
1042-3699/17/© 2016 Elsevier Inc. All rights reserved.

safety movement, described as a culture of error disclosure, apology, and no blame, a supposed contradiction to torts.

There are others who have opined that the threat of torts (malpractice system) is good for patient safety. The concept is that the fear of being sued due to the ever-present possibility that an adverse outcome and/or patient dissatisfaction would result in an allegation of malpractice with the accompanying embarrassment and guilt plus a potential large monetary award would entice a practicing oral and maxillofacial surgeon (OMS) to use safe practice meeting the standard of care. Others claim that the tort system punishes OMSs who have a disregard for practice within the standard of care and the publication of those sanctions and punishments will dissuade any potential patients from seeking care from the identified surgeons. There are little data to prove that the publication of sanctions and punishments will affect the number of patients seeking services from the exposed surgeon.

OMSs are repeatedly reminded during training and in practice to first "do no harm." In many situations, surgical and/or treatment outcomes may be less favorable than desired. When this occurs, there are some people who infer that any unfavorable outcome is in some way, shape, or form an error that is the result of malpractice, a breach of the standard of care, and the fault of the surgeon.

The National Practitioner Data Bank (NPDB) was formed by the US government decades ago. Some of the rationalization for this entity included the concept of patient safety by limitation of privileges and licensure of health care providers being sued, stipulated, or restricted or making a payment to a patient in response to a complaint or claim. Some state licensing/regulatory agencies publish actions taken against licensees for transparency purposes, supposedly to inform potential patients/consumers that the health care provided by the OMS had an adverse action, situation, or result. Again, in theory, potential patients can avoid the clinicians sanctioned, thereby experiencing safer care or management by seeking out or being treated by a health care provider who has not been similarly sanctioned.

Advocates for the tort system of civil liability may make the same allegation. If a health care provider is confronted by an attorney representing a client who is a patient of that provider, he/she may be asked to settle the matter, generally by paying an amount demanded by the attorney. If and when this action is reported to a regulatory agency (licensing board or data bank) and those actions become public, a potential patient may decide to avoid that individual so sanctioned, thereby increasing safety of care for that individual or for the population as a whole.

If a civil lawsuit is filed, there may be public disclosure of the action. In times past, legal counsel may have demanded a large settlement or suit value, into the millions or tens of millions of dollars, generally making the headlines in the press. As the prospective patient population becomes aware of the litigation, they may choose to avoid treatment by the individual named as the defendant.

There are few, if any, data that prove that the tort system, the court of public opinion, the NPDB, the regulatory/licensing agencies, or any other mechanism influenced by these reports results in safer patient care. It may be argued that, when comparing early reports of medical error contributing to from 44,000 to 98,000 deaths in the United States in the 1990s[2] with recent reports of more than 250,000 deaths in the United States due to medical error,[3] we have in fact suffered more deaths in spite of all the patient safety initiatives that have been proposed and integrated over the past 15 years. A confirmation of this suggestion is found in the annual public report of adverse health events in Minnesota, with the number of overall adverse events remaining relatively unchanged over the past 8 years.[4]

RISK MANAGEMENT AND IMPACT ON PATIENT SAFETY
Risk Management

Risk management associated with medical professional liability insurance providers is understood to mean reduction of risk of a claim or lawsuit against a health care provider. It does not generally refer to reduction of the risk of oral and maxillofacial surgical care to the patient being treated.

Many professional liability insurers offer or require participation in courses, seminars, online modules, office inspections, and other mechanisms to manage risk associated with rendering oral and maxillofacial surgical care. The objective of these courses is primarily to manage or reduce the risks associated with OMS care to avoid the possibility of a claim or lawsuit. They also provide information regarding what to do in situations when there may be adverse outcome.

Informed Consent

A highlight and heavily referenced component of risk management is the informed consent process. Required by most regulatory agencies, informed consent is required for most surgical procedures performed by OMSs. The process includes but is not limited to the doctor informing the patient regarding the planned surgical procedures, alternative procedures to those recommended, risks and complications associated with those procedures, the management of complications if they occur, and the risk of declining the recommended treatment.

In some courses, closed claims that have already been settled by litigation, mediation, arbitration, or settlement are used to demonstrate untoward or less than acceptable outcomes from oral and maxillofacial surgical procedures. The presenters describe, from hindsight and retrospective approach, which behaviors may have been used so that the untoward outcome may not have occurred or the claim may not have been filed. This many times hinges on the legibility and completeness of the records for the patient. Although legible, proper, thorough, and complete medical and dental records are good practice, failure to maintain good records is not malpractice. Yet many times the ability to defend a claim is predicated on the status of the records associated with the care rendered to the individual who files the claim.

A comprehensive informed consent process with written, signed, and witnessed informed consent has also become a highly emphasized component of risk management courses. Multiple comprehensive lengthy documents listing any potential untoward outcome or complication may be mandated by medical professional liability companies. Each patient undergoing care provided by an OMS has usually undergone this process, consisting of a diagnosis, treatment plan, list of alternative procedures, potential risks and complications, and recovery, with an emphasis on listing complications with the greatest frequency of occurrence, with the addition of more serious or debilitating outcomes that occur with less frequency. Listing complications on written forms, which are signed by patient and surgeon and witnessed by a third party, assures that, at the least, the patient had completed a component of informed consent. Patients would have the opportunity to make the decision regarding what treatment is best for them and the risks associated with that treatment.

Patient Safety Integrated into Risk Management

The primary objective of patient safety measures is not to minimize risk of a malpractice claim. Patient safety measures are focused on obtaining the most optimal outcome with minimization of adverse risk to the patient undergoing oral and maxillofacial surgical care.

When a claim or lawsuit occurs, there may be little dialogue as to how something could have been done differently to avoid the generally unsatisfactory or unexpected outcome. If a procedure or technique modification should have been considered and, if used, would have avoided or mitigated the untoward outcome, it would be challenging to argue that malpractice did not occur. The surgeon has a responsibility to perform procedures at the level that is accepted as the standard of care by his or her peers. Not all undesirable results are indicative of malpractice. Many untoward outcomes are known risks of a proposed procedure that is performed to treat or cure a patient of currently existing or reasonably predictable anticipated pathology. There is no surgical procedure or operation that can be done without risk. A surgeon cannot control the patient's environment, behavior, negligence, or lack of compliance, which may lead to untoward outcomes as well.

Patient safety is a goal that all surgeons should attempt to obtain. Patient safety measures are techniques and procedures that primarily address a patient's overall well-being associated with the health care rendered. These include identification of recurring or repeated complications that may be avoidable by an alteration in technique. For example, if a particular brand of surgical drill or hand piece is identified as associated with an adverse event, such as overheating, resulting in unexpected adjacent tissue injury (such as a serious burn injury to the perioral skin) by a frequency of incident reports to the surgeons medical professional liability insurance carrier, the carrier could assemble the complaints, identify commonalities, and warn both surgeons and the manufacturer that there was increased risk with the use of that drill. Or if a surgical implant or material were determined defective, unsatisfactory, or associated with unanticipated untoward surgical outcomes, the reports of those outcomes to medical professional liability insurance carrier may result in curbing the use of the material until other studies or evaluations could be performed to determine the safety of those implants. If a particular practice or technique associated with the provision of anesthesia and pain control was determined safer than the standard practice, that information could be presented to OMSs so that they could determine if any changes would be of benefit to the patient population served.

Patient safety measures consist of procedures, such as surgical time outs, preoperative and postoperative "brief "discussions, comprehensive presurgical and preanesthesia evaluations, and checklists, including airway assessment and medical assessment and American Society of Anesthesiologists classification. Patient safety measures also include but are not limited to office anesthesia evaluation certifications; qualified dental, surgical, and anesthesia assistants; and emergency drills. These are extra measures, many times in addition to what is considered standards of care, to potentially reduce the risk of adverse outcome.

THE MALPRACTICE TORTS SYSTEM COMPARED WITH DISCLOSURE AND ADMISSION
Anatomy of a Malpractice Claim

A 21-year-old patient is referred to an OMS by a general dentist with an evaluate-and-treat request for impacted third molars. The referring dentist indicates that he/she feels that the teeth should be removed, but the decision will be made by the surgeon and the patient. There are 5-mm periodontal pockets on the distal aspect of all 4 second molars. The teeth are submerged but communicate with the oral cavity. The patient has a high caries index with dental restorations on first and second molars in all 4 quadrants due to caries.

The surgeon advises removal of all the third molars under general anesthesia. Informed consent is rendered with a video presentation, personal conversation, and discussion, and the informed consent is signed and witnessed. The patient returns in 2 weeks at her convenience for the removal of the teeth under general anesthesia.

The procedure is performed without complication. The anesthetic is safely administered. The teeth are surgically removed with standard acceptable procedure with buccal incision, tooth sectioning, and elevation. The procedure takes 20 minutes to perform. There were no variations of standard technique, challenges, or clinical complications with the procedure.

The surgeon phones the patient 1 day postoperatively. To his surprise, the patient reports that the entire right side of the tongue is numb. She reports that the left side felt the same way until approximately 4 hours after the procedure. The surgeon asks the patient to report to his practice. She complies. He confirms that the right half of the tongue is in fact numb. The surgeon reports this complication to his medical professional liability carrier. The claims analyst records the discussion but does not assign defense counsel because the patient has not threatened a lawsuit.

The patient is referred to a microneurosurgeon who evaluates the patient over time and sees no recovery of sensation for 3 months. He then offers nerve surgery in hopes of recovery for the patient. The procedure is performed. The nerve surgeon reveals that the lingual nerve, although intact, appeared "scarred." The patient reports no recovery of feeling in the right tongue in the 12 months after nerve repair. She decides to sue her OMS for malpractice. The OMS is served with a complaint alleging malpractice by the patient's malpractice attorney.

At this point the tort system kicks in. The OMS is generally advised not to discuss the situation with the patient any further. Defense counsel is assigned. All communication from this point forward is through legal counsel. The patient is distressed and feels that her surgeon was negligent because the patient's and plaintiff attorney's expert witness has said so.

The OMS feels that the lingual nerve injury is a known risk of the procedure and that the patient was fully informed and signed a document that stated that fact. He knows that his surgical technique was standard and accepted. He made no mistakes.

Both sides do not wish to concede. The patient's demand for settlement approaches $500,000. The OMS is insured for $1 million.

In the tort system, if no settlement can be reached, this case may go to trial. To do so takes considerable time (several months to perhaps a year or 2) to be litigated. There are significant costs associated with the legal process. The jury is left to decide who, if anyone, should concede.

Anatomy of Disclosure and Admission

The same scenario occurs until the point of the lawsuit being filed. If the surgeon is employed by a health care organization, hospital, or large group practice, the risk management team may take control of this situation. Oral and maxillofacial surgical practices in general do not have the opportunity to use a program similar to the Communication and Optimal Resolution program[5] as proposed by the Agency for Healthcare Research and Quality. Although self-insured entities may determine that there may be many benefits of this type of program, including cost savings, compared with traditional management of medical/dental professional liability claims, it is not currently available to OMSs in private practice.

Many claims are billing disputes. Defense verdicts for OMS malpractice claims litigated in court have exceeded 90% for many years. This can be offered as proof that many malpractice claims are frivolous in the eyes of juries that deliberate them. Some claims, however, are still won by the plaintiff, even when the jury opines that no malpractice occurred, but they thought that the plaintiff should be compensated for pain and suffering.

Without the knowledge and expertise of experienced risk management personnel, an OMS unfamiliar with how a malpractice claim is managed may compromise their claim of no negligence by attempting to settle this situation on his own. It is certain that there would be high likelihood of missteps that could result in significant risk to personal assets if the confrontation and untoward outcome are litigated without counsel. Communication and offers of aid could lead to significant financial loss even in a situation where the standard of care has not been breached.

There is a wide range of jury awards or settlements made with lingual nerve injury. What is an acceptable compensation? Variations may be associated with jurisdiction, degree of injury, cost of subsequent care, impact on ability to perform normal oral function, employability, presence of pain, and numerous other factors.

To some degree, although the communication and optimal resolution program may reduce the cost of attorneys, experts, court proceedings, judges, discovery, trials, time away from work, and other entities, does it reduce the amount of the compensation or settlement to the aggrieved party? Can it be assured that the overall cost of the events will be reduced, thereby reducing the cost of health care in the United States?

These questions must be addressed and researched before the concept of saying "I'm sorry" when an injury has occurred but there is no demonstrable malpractice. Surgical procedures will always be associated with risk.

Exceptional surgeons sustain complications and untoward outcomes. The occurrence of complications does not mean that a procedure is unnecessary or that it was done wrong. There would have to be significant tort reform, caps on malpractice awards, establishment of patient compensation systems, limits of settlement amounts, and some ground rules in the OMS environment for any chance of success with this endeavor.

Until that time, medical professional liability companies should stress the patient safety pursuit by the oral and maxillofacial surgery profession to reduce, if possible, the number of complications that can occur with OMS procedures.

REFERENCES

1. Clinton HR, Obama B. Making patient safety the centerpiece of medical liability reform. N Engl J Med 2006;354(21):2205–8.
2. Kohn LT. To err is human building a safer health system. National Academy Press; 2000. Executive Summary 1.
3. Makary MA, Daniel M. Medical error-the third leading cause of death in the US. BMJ 2016;353:i2139.
4. Annual Public Report, Adverse Health Events in Minnesota, February 2016. p. 9. Available at: www.health.state.mn.us/patientsafety. Accessed January 24, 2017.
5. Communication and Optimal Resolution (CANDOR) US Department of Health and Human Services, Agency for Healthcare Research and Quality. Available at: http://www.ahrq.gov/professionals/quality-patient-safety/patient-safety-resources/resources/candor/index.html. Accessed January 24, 2017.

Quality Improvement and Reporting Systems
What the Oral and Maxillofacial Surgeon Should Know

Justine S. Moe, DDS, MD, Shelly Abramowicz, DMD, MPH,
Steven M. Roser, DMD, MD*

KEYWORDS

- Patient safety • Safety program • Safety culture • Risk assessment • Medical error
- Surgical time-out • Surgical checklist

KEY POINTS

- Patient safety is a discipline in health care that aims to reduce the incidence and impact of adverse events.
- A safety program in the OMS practice can be used to implement standardized patient safety practices, incident reporting, and adverse event analysis.
- The surgical checklist and surgical time-out can prevent perioperative adverse events in OMS.
- A standardized tool for risk assessment and internal and external benchmarking is currently lacking in OMS.

INTRODUCTION

The Hippocratic "primum non nocere" is a fundamental principle in medicine and oral and maxillofacial surgery (OMS). Paradoxically, health care is a highly hazardous industry, and surgery is inherently risky for patients.[1] A recent review[2] found that 1 in every 150 inpatients dies as a consequence of an adverse event (AE) and nearly two-thirds of in-hospital events are associated with surgical care. Medical error is now estimated to be the third leading cause of death in the United States, killing approximately 250,000 people each year.[3]

OMS is not immune to risk. Between 1988 and 1999, a total of 136 anesthesia claims were managed by the American Association of Oral and Maxillofacial Surgeons National Insurance Company including 37 claims relating to death or brain damage[4] (**Table 1**). Promoting patient safety should thus be a priority within OMS.

DEFINING PATIENT SAFETY

In 2000, the Institute of Medicine[5] published the report, "To Err is Human: Building a Safer Health System," which launched the modern patient safety movement. Following the report, the federal Agency for Healthcare Research and Quality (AHRQ) was directed to lead the national effort to combat medical errors and to improve patient safety through multiple initiatives.[6] Patient safety has since developed into a discipline that applies

Disclosure: The authors have nothing to disclose.
Division of Oral and Maxillofacial Surgery, Department of Surgery, Emory University School of Medicine, 1365B Clifton Road, Atlanta, GA 30322, USA
* Corresponding author.
E-mail address: sroser@emory.edu

Oral Maxillofacial Surg Clin N Am 29 (2017) 229–238
http://dx.doi.org/10.1016/j.coms.2016.12.011
1042-3699/17/© 2017 Elsevier Inc. All rights reserved.

Table 1 Anesthesia claims from 1988 to 1999	
Vein/nerve injuries	52
Death or brain damage	37
Falls	6
Inadequate anesthesia	7
Premature discharge	3
Allergic reactions	3
Stormy emergence	5
Arrhythmia/resuscitation	6
Acute myocardial infarction	2
Other	15
Total anesthesia claims	136

From Deegan AE. Anesthesia morbidity and mortality, 1988-1999: claims statistics from AAOMS National Insurance Company. Anesth Prog 2001;48(3):90; with permission.

safety science methods with the goal of achieving a trustworthy system of health care delivery.[7]

The National Patient Safety Foundation[8] defines patient safety as "the avoidance, prevention and amelioration of adverse outcomes or injuries stemming from the processes of healthcare." Errors in safety are reduced by redesigning systems of care using human factors principles.[7] In OMS, accepting a paradigm shift in which patient safety is given a high priority as an outcome that is tracked, measured, and benchmarked over time is paramount in optimizing patient outcomes.

PROMOTING A SAFETY CULTURE

Cultivating a "culture of safety" is necessary to establish the foundation for a successful safety program in OMS. Safety culture is defined as "the product of individual and group values, attitudes, perceptions, skills and patterns of behavior which lead to commitment, style and ability in the management of the health and safety of an organization."[9,10]

The traditional "culture of blame" is pervasive in health care and surgery. It focuses on determining fault and disciplining the offender. The fear of reprimand inherently leads to chronic underreporting of adverse effects, thus limiting the possibility of learning from error.[1,11] In contrast, a culture of safety promotes nonpunitive responses to AEs. It focuses on preventing future injury and improving clinical outcomes rather than on individual mistakes.[11,12]

To establish a safety culture, patient safety should be a priority corporate objective and should be understood to be the shared responsibility of all staff members.[5] Rather than viewing errors as unique and sometimes tragic events, the focus should be to continually improve the organizational safety system design and practices.[5] The importance of a culture of safety has been recognized in dentistry[13–15] and other surgical specialties.

IMPLEMENTING A SAFETY PROGRAM

OMS can learn from the success of highly reliable industries including aviation, nuclear power, oil and gas, and the military, all of which have developed sophisticated safety systems for minimizing errors and accidents.[16] The positive effects on clinical outcomes, patient safety, and efficacy of care following changes in health care safety practices have been widely reported.[17–23]

Fundamental components of a safety program include implementing practices to minimize risk and developing a systematic approach for the management of AEs.

Minimizing Risks

Patient safety interventions designed to prevent harm were first described by the Institute of Medicine[5] (**Box 1**). The AHRQ developed evidence-based patient safety practices aimed to reduce the probability of AEs over a broad range of diseases and procedures.[24] These practices were recently categorized as "strongly encouraged" and "encouraged" based on critical analysis of available data[25] (**Box 2**). Patient safety practices have been implemented at various levels of health care and have been endorsed by the National Quality Forum.[26]

Managing Adverse Events

A systematic approach for managing AEs is important for organizations to continuously modify safety systems to allow for future risk reduction. Key components include practices for incident reporting and AE analysis.

Incident reporting

To date, the detection of AEs occurs primarily by voluntary reporting. Consequently, most AEs are not tracked, with only an estimated 10% to 20% of errors ever reported.[27] In OMS, the most common sources of information regarding AEs are published case reports, ethical complaints, court claims, and voluntary anonymous reports by professionals or patients. There is thus a need in OMS for active surveillance, systematic notification, and recording of AEs.

Many reporting systems have been described. The "trigger tool system" developed by the

---

Box 1
Examples of patient safety interventions to minimize medical error

1. Incorporating user-centered designs
   a. Clearly written set of instructions on equipment describing how to change the settings

2. Avoiding reliance on memory
   a. Establish the usual dose of a medication as the default setting in an electronic order entry system

3. Attending to work safety
   a. Establish "safe zones" where nurses can prepare or administer medications without distractions

4. Avoiding reliance on vigilance
   a. Use of the presurgical checklist

5. Training for team collaboration
   a. Training programs for interprofessional communication and collaboration to promote culture of safety

6. Involving patients in their care
   a. Include patients and families when making decisions about treatments, offer educational information, and prepare discharge plans

7. Anticipating the unexpected
   a. Involve front-line users in pilot testing before widespread implementation of new processes and technologies, such as changing from a paper record to an electronic health care record

8. Designing for recovery
   a. Simulate equipment failures to hone provider skills, identify equipment vulnerabilities, and evaluate alternative approaches or procedures

9. Improving access to accurate, timely information
   a. Easy access to drug formularies, evidence-based practice protocols, patient records, laboratory reports, and medication administration records at the point of care

Adapted from Barnsteiner J. Teaching the culture of safety. Online J Issues Nurs 2011;16(3):5; with permission.

Institute for Healthcare Improvement[28] is a systematic retrospective review of randomly selected medical records. Experienced personnel screen records for triggers, which are events or circumstances that may indicate a health care–related injury. All AEs that are subsequently identified are recorded.

The use of trigger tools has been shown to identify previously undetected AEs and has been used to guide quality improvement efforts.[29] In addition, a common terminology and classification schema of safety events have been proposed by the World Health Organization (WHO)[30] and by the Joint Commission (JC)[31] to allow for standardized reporting.

In dentistry, Maramaldi and colleagues[32] developed a preliminary inventory of dental AEs that may be used to track, prevent, and mitigate these events. Kalenderian and colleagues[33] described a dental clinic trigger tool to improve the identification of AEs. In OMS, AE reporting systems have not been developed at the time of this publication.

Adverse event analysis

Following the occurrence of an AE, a structured method of identifying contributing or causal factors is necessary to implement changes aimed at preventing future harm. Root cause analysis (RCA) is an error analysis tool for data collection and event reconstruction through record review and participant interviews[34] (**Fig. 1**). The RCA data can be used by a multidisciplinary team to identify how and why the AE occurred and thus work to eliminate latent errors within a system.[35] RCA is one of the most widely used approaches to improving patient safety.

Health care failure mode and effects analysis (HFMEA) is a prospective analysis tool developed by the Department of Veteran Affairs that uses reported data to prevent similar events in similar procedures.[36–38] It involves the analysis of a process by a multidisciplinary team to identify potential problems at each step and to design and implement changes to reduce or prevent error. HFMEA

Box 2
AHRQ patient safety practices

Strongly encouraged patient safety practices

- Preoperative checklists and anesthesia checklists to prevent operative and postoperative events.
- Bundles that include checklists to prevent central line–associated bloodstream infections.
- Interventions to reduce urinary catheter use, including catheter reminders, stop orders, or nurse-initiated removal protocols.
- Bundles that include head-of-bed elevation, sedation vacations, oral care with chlorhexidine, and subglottic-suctioning endotracheal tubes to prevent ventilator-associated pneumonia.
- Hand hygiene.
- "Do Not Use" list for hazardous abbreviations.
- Multicomponent interventions to reduce pressure ulcers.
- Barrier precautions to prevent health care–associated infections.
- Use of real-time ultrasound for central line placement.
- Interventions to improve prophylaxis for venous thromboembolisms.

Encouraged patient safety practices

- Multicomponent interventions to reduce falls.
- Use of clinical pharmacists to reduce adverse drug events.
- Documentation of patient preferences for life-sustaining treatment.
- Obtaining informed consent to improve patients' understanding of the potential risks of procedures.
- Team training.
- Medication reconciliation.
- Practices to reduce radiation exposure from fluoroscopy and computed tomography scans.
- Use of surgical outcome measurements and report cards, such as the American College of Surgeons National Surgical Quality Improvement Program.
- Rapid response systems.
- Use of complementary methods for detecting adverse events/medical errors to monitor for patient safety problems.
- Computerized provider order entry.
- Use of simulation exercises in patient safety efforts.

From Agency for Healthcare Research and Quality. Making Health Care Safer II: An Updated Critical Analysis of the Evidence for Patient Safety Practices. 2013. Available at: http://www.ahrq.gov/research/findings/evidence-based-reports/ptsafetyuptp.html. Accessed August 8, 2016; with permission.

---

is used by many health care systems on a voluntary basis. For example, HFMEA implementation is a component of the Institute for Healthcare Improvement and Centers for Medicare and Medicaid Services improvement programs and is one method of complying with JC accreditation. AE analysis tools for OMS have not been reported at the time of this publication.

ASSESSMENT OF SAFETY PROGRAMS

Regular assessment of the safety program of a health care system is important to monitor its efficacy and is often mandated by directives or regulatory requirements.

Self-Assessment Tools

Safety culture self-assessment tools are structured self-report surveys that evaluate safety interventions and programs, identify areas for improvement, and raise awareness about patient safety.[1] Multiple self-assessment tools exist and are intended for use by health care providers, managerial personnel, organizational leadership, and multidisciplinary teams.[39,40]

One survey from the Voluntary Hospitals of America and American Hospital Association lists key safety aspects (eg, promoting a nonpunitive culture) and asks respondents to indicate the extent to which the activity has been implemented

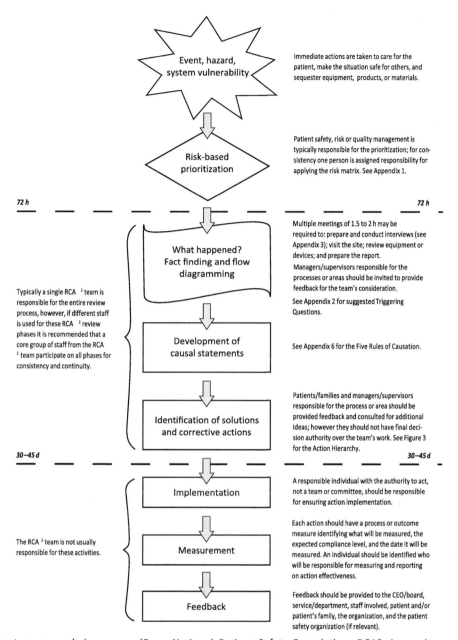

Fig. 1. Root cause analysis process. (*From* National Patient Safety Foundation. RCA2: improving root cause analyses and actions to prevent harm. Boston, MA: National Patient Safety Foundation; 2015. Available at http://www.npsf.org/?RCA2.)

throughout the organization on a five-point Likert scale.[41] The Accreditation Council for Graduate Medical Education developed the Clinical Learning Environment Review program to evaluate and improve the learning environment in teaching hospitals.[42]

Although safety culture assessment tools have been studied extensively, there is currently limited evidence regarding their validity. Challenges include comparing tools that are highly diverse in terms of general characteristics, dimensions covered, and psychometrics performed.[43] The choice of tool by different health care systems also varies depending on its intended use and target population.[1] No data on safety culture assessment tools in OMS have been reported at the time of this publication.

Benchmarking

Internal and external benchmarking are important processes in standardizing health care delivery.

The self-assessment tools described previously may be used for this purpose. The AHRQ *Hospital Survey on Patient Safety Culture* allowed hospitals to compare their patient safety culture survey results with those of other hospitals, with the most recent report[44] listing responses from 622 hospitals and 196,462 hospital staff.

Benchmarked data are also collected by health care organizations, consumers, and insurance companies. It is used by health care consumers in choosing health care delivery organizations and by the organizations in quality improvement and competitor analysis efforts.[1,45] For example, the National Committee for Quality Assurance, a not-for-profit organization, publishes the Quality Compass, which provides national, regional, and individual health plan data on performance and customer satisfaction.[46] The goal of sharing data on medical error and patient safety within and between organizations, nationally and internationally is to achieve more reliable health care systems.

In dentistry, Ramoni and colleagues[47] published the first use of the AHRQ Medical Office Survey on Patient Safety Culture at three dental schools, highlighting clinical and educational priorities for improving the safety of care in dental school clinics. Leong and colleagues[48] reported that the AHRQ Medical Office Survey on Patient Safety Culture administered to faculty, students, and support staff members in the clinics of seven U.S. dental schools showed patient safety attitudes of dental school participants were higher than those of their hospital counterparts. No data for benchmarking patient safety in OMS were available at the time of this publication.

EXTERNAL DRIVERS OF SAFETY

Patient safety is addressed through a collaborative effort of many stakeholders including health care providers, medical technology companies, health care institutions, clinical bodies (eg, the American Medical Association), private payors, regulatory groups, state health departments, federal governing bodies (eg, the U.S. Department of Health and Human Services), and global organizations (eg, the WHO). As such, incentives to develop patient safety programs arise from many external drivers.

The Centers for Medicare and Medicaid Services have linked the performance on quality indicators, such as central line infections, with hospital payment.[49] The JC has issued safety standards necessary for accreditation, including National Patient Safety Goals and handoff communication guidelines.[50] "The Universal Protocol for Preventing Wrong-Site, Wrong-Procedure, Wrong-Person Surgery"[51] introduced by the JC mandates standard perioperative practices to ensure correct patient identity, correct scheduled procedure, and correct surgical site.

The National Surgical Quality Improvement Program (NSQIP) of the American College of Surgeons (ACS)[52] has become central to the organization's national surgical quality improvement agenda. The foundation for NSQIP was borne in the mid-1980s when a U.S. government mandate was issued in response to a high rate of perioperative mortality and surgical complications among the 133 Veterans Administration (VA) hospitals. It called for the annual reporting of surgical outcomes, adjusted for the severity of patients' illnesses, with the goal of minimizing perioperative complications in VA hospitals.[53]

From this clinical database, parameters of risk adjustment were established that, in 1994, allowed for risk-adjusted outcome comparison among VA hospitals. NSQIP was highly successful, reducing postoperative 30-day mortality and morbidity by 47% and 43%, respectively, from 1991 to 2006.[54] The program was adopted by ACS and was initiated nationally as ACS NSQIP in 2004.

The ACS NSQIP database currently provides risk-adjusted surgical outcome measures for participating hospitals and is used for performance improvement of surgical morbidity and mortality.[53] In addition to its standard program, ACS NSQIP offers multiple participation options to accommodate all hospital types including a procedure-targeted program, a small and rural program, and a pediatric program.[55]

There currently is a lack of any means of assessing risk-adjusted surgical outcome measures in OMS for internal or external benchmarking. Although comparable otolaryngology operations, such as facial fracture repair, are included in NSQIP, specific OMS procedures, such as dental extractions and implants, are not. Furthermore, the foundations necessary for such a database for OMS are not currently in place, because it requires a broad-based patient reporting system to be established.

FUTURE DIRECTION

OMS has lagged behind the medical field in making the public aware of its attention to patient safety. There is a paucity of research in the area of patient safety and there are currently no published organizational guidelines for patient safety in OMS.

The current NSQIP database may be ineffective in predicting outcomes in OMS. For example, a retrospective cohort study[56] found the ACS-NSQIP surgical risk calculator to be ineffective in predicting postoperative complications in patients undergoing microvascular head and neck reconstruction.

A potential area of contribution by OMS may be to develop a database of risk-adjusted surgical outcomes specific to hospital-based OMS procedures that may be used in conjunction with the NSQIP database. In addition, a patient safety program should include office-based procedures to capture most patients treated by OMS. The American Association of Oral and Maxillofacial Surgeons–sponsored OMS Quality Outcomes Registry was being piloted at the time of this publication as a means to collect and report OMS outcomes from electronic health records for benchmarking and tracking performance.[57] This database may be an appropriate platform to track patient safety practices in the OMS office.

Two currently accepted patient safety practices that may be useful for adoption in the OMS office-based practice include implementation of the surgical checklist and the surgical time-out. Long used in aviation, the surgical checklist has emerged as a practical and effective tool for developing a safer health care environment. The goal of the checklist is to present critical tasks as a list, a format that simplifies understanding and recall of information, creates reliable evaluations, reduces the occurrence of errors of omission, and ensures the use of best practices.[58]

Surgical checklists have been widely implemented and have been shown to reduce perioperative complications.[59] Standard surgical checklists have been made available by the JC[60] and the WHO[61] (**Fig. 2**). The WHO Safe Surgery Saves Lives Study Group found that a perioperative surgical safety checklist was associated with an absolute risk reduction in 30-day morbidity and mortality of 4.0% and 0.7%, respectively.[62] The Surgical Patient Safety System multidisciplinary checklist used from admission to discharge was associated with an absolute risk reduction in surgical complications and in-hospital mortality of 10.6% and 0.7%, respectively.[63,64] Bock and colleagues[65] found the implementation of surgical safety checklists to be associated with a decrease in all-cause 90-day mortality and hospital length of stay.

In dentistry, a checklist to standardize the process of dental implant placement has been described.[66] A standardized checklist in OMS has not been developed at the time of this publication.

The pause, or surgical time-out before incision, is the final recapitulation and reassurance of accurate patient identity, surgical site, and planned procedure.[67,68] An extended time-out may also include quality parameters or a formal briefing for the entire surgical team. The time-out is an integral component of the JC "Universal Protocol" and is

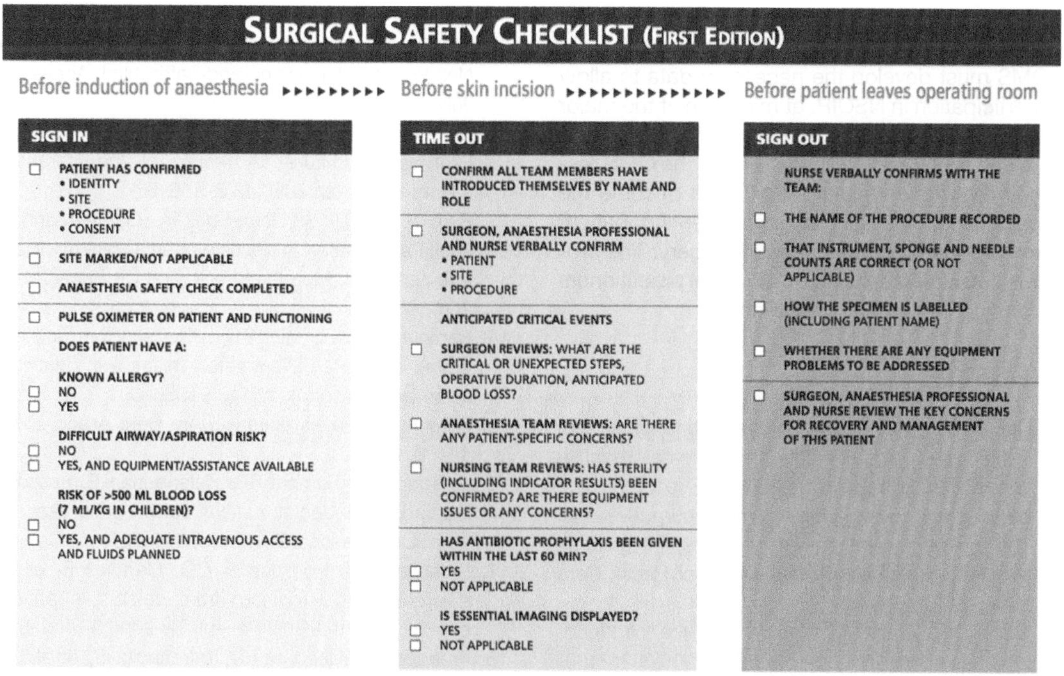

SURGICAL SAFETY CHECKLIST (FIRST EDITION)

Before induction of anaesthesia ▸▸▸▸▸▸▸▸▸ Before skin incision ▸▸▸▸▸▸▸▸▸▸▸▸▸▸ Before patient leaves operating room

SIGN IN

☐ PATIENT HAS CONFIRMED
• IDENTITY
• SITE
• PROCEDURE
• CONSENT

☐ SITE MARKED/NOT APPLICABLE

☐ ANAESTHESIA SAFETY CHECK COMPLETED

☐ PULSE OXIMETER ON PATIENT AND FUNCTIONING

DOES PATIENT HAVE A:

KNOWN ALLERGY?
☐ NO
☐ YES

DIFFICULT AIRWAY/ASPIRATION RISK?
☐ NO
☐ YES, AND EQUIPMENT/ASSISTANCE AVAILABLE

RISK OF >500 ML BLOOD LOSS (7 ML/KG IN CHILDREN)?
☐ NO
☐ YES, AND ADEQUATE INTRAVENOUS ACCESS AND FLUIDS PLANNED

TIME OUT

☐ CONFIRM ALL TEAM MEMBERS HAVE INTRODUCED THEMSELVES BY NAME AND ROLE

☐ SURGEON, ANAESTHESIA PROFESSIONAL AND NURSE VERBALLY CONFIRM
• PATIENT
• SITE
• PROCEDURE

ANTICIPATED CRITICAL EVENTS

☐ SURGEON REVIEWS: WHAT ARE THE CRITICAL OR UNEXPECTED STEPS, OPERATIVE DURATION, ANTICIPATED BLOOD LOSS?

☐ ANAESTHESIA TEAM REVIEWS: ARE THERE ANY PATIENT-SPECIFIC CONCERNS?

☐ NURSING TEAM REVIEWS: HAS STERILITY (INCLUDING INDICATOR RESULTS) BEEN CONFIRMED? ARE THERE EQUIPMENT ISSUES OR ANY CONCERNS?

HAS ANTIBIOTIC PROPHYLAXIS BEEN GIVEN WITHIN THE LAST 60 MIN?
☐ YES
☐ NOT APPLICABLE

IS ESSENTIAL IMAGING DISPLAYED?
☐ YES
☐ NOT APPLICABLE

SIGN OUT

NURSE VERBALLY CONFIRMS WITH THE TEAM:

☐ THE NAME OF THE PROCEDURE RECORDED

☐ THAT INSTRUMENT, SPONGE AND NEEDLE COUNTS ARE CORRECT (OR NOT APPLICABLE)

☐ HOW THE SPECIMEN IS LABELLED (INCLUDING PATIENT NAME)

☐ WHETHER THERE ARE ANY EQUIPMENT PROBLEMS TO BE ADDRESSED

☐ SURGEON, ANAESTHESIA PROFESSIONAL AND NURSE REVIEW THE KEY CONCERNS FOR RECOVERY AND MANAGEMENT OF THIS PATIENT

Fig. 2. WHO surgical checklist. (*From* World Health Organization. WHO surgical safety checklist and implementation manual. Available at: http://www.who.int/patientsafety/safesurgery/ss_checklist/en/. Accessed August 8, 2016; with permission.)

important in identifying "near miss events."[69] It helps to mitigate the hierarchal style in the operating room and places the responsibility of error prevention on the entire team.[68,70]

In a cross-sectional study of operating room personnel including surgeons, anesthetists, nurse anesthetists, and operating room nurses, 38% of respondents had experienced uncertainty of patient identity, 81% had experienced uncertainty of the surgical site, and 60% had prepared for the wrong procedure.[71]

The role of the time-out in reducing wrong-sided surgeries has not been proven.[68,70] However, the time-out improves communication between team members and has not been found to disrupt workflow.[68] Implementation of the surgical time-out in the OMS practice has the potential to reduce wrong site surgery, including extraction of the incorrect tooth.

SUMMARY

Health care is an inherently dangerous environment and patient safety should be an explicit goal of OMS. Important components of a safety program include a nonpunitive safety culture, the implementation of patient safety practices, standardized incident reporting and AE analysis, regular self-assessment, and internal and external benchmarking. Implementation of a safety program requires the strong commitment of leadership and the engagement and empowerment of all employees.

OMS must develop the necessary data to allow for participation in NSQIP, at minimum at the major medical centers. The fundamentals of patient safety practices should be a required part of the OMS residency didactic curriculum. OMS can become the model dental specialty by implementing patient safety programs for office-based surgery. The programs could then be used by all dental practitioners performing oral surgery in the office.

REFERENCES

1. Nieva VF, Sorra J. Safety culture assessment: a tool for improving patient safety in healthcare organizations. Qual Saf Health Care 2003;12(Suppl 2):17–23.
2. de Vries EN, Ramrattan MA, Smorenburg SM, et al. The incidence and nature of in-hospital adverse events: a systematic review. Qual Saf Health Care 2008;17(3):216–23.
3. Makary MA, Daniel M. Medical error-the third leading cause of death in the US. BMJ 2016;353:i2139.
4. Deegan AE. Anesthesia morbidity and mortality, 1988-1999: claims statistics from AAOMS National Insurance Company. Anesth Prog 2001;48(3):89–92.
5. Kohn LT, Corrigan JM, Donaldson MS. Committee on Quality of Health Care in America, Institute of Medicine. To err is human: building a safer health system. Washington, DC: The National Academies Press; 2000.
6. Agency for Healthcare Research and Quality. Quality and patient safety. Available at: http://www.ahrq.gov/professionals/quality-patient-safety/index.html. Accessed August 8, 2016.
7. Emanuel L, Berwick D, Conway J, et al. What exactly is patient safety?. In: Henriksen K, Battles JB, Keyes MA, et al, editors. Advances in patient safety: new directions and alternative approaches, vol. 1 Rockville (MD): Agency for Healthcare Research and Quality; 2008. Available at: https://www.ncbi.nlm.nih.gov/books/NBK43629/. Accessed August 8, 2016.
8. National Patient Safety Foundation. Patient safety dictionary. Available at: http://www.npsf.org/?page=dictionarynz. Accessed July 17, 2016.
9. Health and Safety Commission Advisory Committee on the Safety of Nuclear Installations. Organizing for safety: third report of the ACSNI study group on human factors. Sudbury (Canada): HSE Books; 1993.
10. The Institution of Engineering and Technology. Safety Culture: Health and Safety Briefing No. 07, February 2015. Available at: www.theiet.org/factfiles/health/hsb07-page.cfm?type=pdf. Accessed August 8, 2016.
11. Barnsteiner J. Teaching the culture of safety. Online J Issues Nurs 2011;16(3):5. Available at: http://www.nursingworld.org/MainMenuCategories/ANAMarketplace/ANAPeriodicals/OJIN/TableofContents/Vol-16-2011/No3-Sept-2011/Teaching-and-Safety.html. Accessed July 17, 2016.
12. Sammer CE, Lykens K, Singh KP, et al. What is patient safety culture? A review of the literature. J Nurs Scholarsh 2010;42(2):156–65.
13. Perea-Pérez B, Santiago-Sáez A, García-Marín F, et al. Patient safety in dentistry: dental care risk management plan. Med Oral Patol Oral Cir Bucal 2011; 16(6):e805–9.
14. Ramoni RB, Walji MF, White J, et al. From good to better: toward a patient safety initiative in dentistry. J Am Dent Assoc 2012;143(9):956–60.
15. Sinykin SG. Patient safety. J Am Dent Assoc 2013; 144(1):18–9.
16. Obadan EM, Ramoni RB, Kalenderian E. Lessons learned from dental patient safety case reports. J Am Dent Assoc 2015;146(5):318–26.
17. Pronovost PJ, Holzmueller CG, Martinez E, et al. A practical tool to learn from defects in patient care. Jt Comm J Qual Patient Saf 2006;32:102–8.
18. Pronovost P, Needham D, Berenholtz S, et al. An intervention to decrease catheter-related bloodstream infections in the ICU. N Engl J Med 2006; 355:2725–32.

19. Pronovost P, Weast B, Schwarz M, et al. Medication reconciliation: a practical tool to reduce the risk of medication errors. J Crit Care 2003;18:201–5.

20. Resar R, Pronovost P, Haraden C, et al. Using a bundle approach to improve ventilator care processes and reduce ventilator-associated pneumonia. Jt Comm J Qual Patient Saf 2005;31:243–8.

21. Levy MM, Pronovost PJ, Dellinger RP, et al. Sepsis change bundles: converting guidelines into meaningful change in behavior and clinical outcome. Crit Care Med 2004;32(Suppl):S595–7.

22. Leape LL, Cullen DJ, Clapp MD, et al. Pharmacist participation on physician rounds and adverse drug events in the intensive care unit. JAMA 1999; 282:267–70.

23. Rodriguez-Paz JM, Mark LJ, Herzer KR, et al. A novel process for introducing a new intraoperative program: a multidisciplinary paradigm for mitigating hazards and improving patient safety. Anesth Analg 2009;108(1):202–10.

24. Shojania KG, Duncan BW, McDonald KM, et al. Making health care safer: a critical analysis of patient safety practices. Rockville (MD): Agency for Healthcare Research and Quality; 2001.

25. Agency for Healthcare Research and Quality. Making Health Care Safer II: an updated critical analysis of the evidence for patient safety practices. 2013. Available at: http://www.ahrq.gov/research/findings/evidence-based-reports/ptsafetyuptp.html. Accessed August 8, 2016.

26. National Quality Forum. National voluntary consensus standards for patient safety. Available at: http://www.qualityforum.org/projects/patient_safety_measures.aspx. Accessed August 8, 2016.

27. Institute of Healthcare Improvement. Adverse drug events per 1,000 doses. Available at: http://www.ihi.org/resources/Pages/Measures/ADEsper1000Doses.aspx. Accessed August 8, 2016.

28. Institute of Healthcare Improvement. Introduction to trigger tools for identifying adverse events. Available at: http://www.ihi.org/resources/Pages/Tools/IntrotoTriggerToolsforIdentifyingAEs.aspx. Accessed July 17, 2016.

29. Mull HJ, Brennan CW, Folkes T, et al. Identifying previously undetected harm: piloting the institute for healthcare improvement's global trigger tool in the Veterans' Health Administration. Qual Manag Health Care 2015;24(3):140–6.

30. Runciman W, Hibbert P, Thomson R, et al. Towards an international classification for patient safety: key concepts and terms. Int J Qual Health Care 2009; 21(1):18–26.

31. Chang A, Schyve PM, Croteau RJ, et al. The JCAHO patient safety event taxonomy: a standardized terminology and classification schema for near misses and adverse events. Int J Qual Health Care 2005; 17(2):95–105.

32. Maramaldi P, Walji MF, White J, et al. How dental team members describe adverse events. J Am Dent Assoc 2016;147(10):803–11.

33. Kalenderian E, Walji MF, Tavares A, et al. An adverse event trigger tool in dentistry: a new methodology for measuring harm in the dental office. J Am Dent Assoc 2013;144(7):808–14.

34. National Patient Safety Foundation. RCA^2: improving root cause analyses and actions to prevent harm. Boston: National Patient Safety Foundation; 2016. Available at: http://www.npsf.org/?page=RCA2. Accessed August 8, 2016.

35. Agency for Healthcare Research and Quality. Root cause analysis. Available at: https://psnet.ahrq.gov/primers/primer/10/root-cause-analysis. Accessed July 17, 2016.

36. Spath PL. Using failure mode and effects analysis to improve patient safety. AORN J 2003;78(1):16–37.

37. DeRosier J, Stalhandske E, Bagian JP, et al. Using health care failure mode and effect analysis: the VA national center for patient safety's prospective risk analysis system. Jt Comm J Qual Improv 2002; 28(5):248–67.

38. Reiling J. Safe design of healthcare facilities. Qual Saf Health Care 2006;15(Suppl 1):34–40.

39. Scott T, Mannion R, Davies H, et al. The quantitative measurement of organizational culture in health care: a review of the available instruments. Health Serv Res 2003;38(3):923–45.

40. Singla AK, Kitch BT, Weissman JS, et al. Assessing patient safety culture: a review and synthesis of the measurement tools. J Patient Saf 2006;2:105–15.

41. American Hospital Association. Strategies for leadership: a hospital self-assessment inventory. Available at: http://www.aha.org/content/00-10/assessment.pdf. Accessed July 17, 2016.

42. Bump GM, Coots N, Liberi CA, et al. Comparing trainee and staff perceptions of patient safety culture. Acad Med 2017;92(1):116–22.

43. Colla JB, Bracken AC, Kinney LM, et al. Measuring patient safety climate: a review of surveys. Qual Saf Health Care 2005;14(5):364–6.

44. Sorra J, Famolaro T, Dyer N, et al. Hospital survey on patient safety culture: 2009 comparative database report. Rockville (MD): Agency for Healthcare Research and Quality; 2009.

45. Agency for Healthcare Research and Quality. CAHPS: surveys and tools to advance patient-centered care. Available at: http://www.ahrq.gov/cahps/index.html. Accessed July 17, 2016.

46. National Committee for Quality Assurance. HEDIS and Quality Compass. Available at: http://www.ncqa.org/hedis-quality-measurement/what-is-hedis. Accessed July 17, 2016.

47. Ramoni R, Walji MF, Tavares A, et al. Open wide: looking into the safety culture of dental school clinics. J Dent Educ 2014;78(5):745–56.

48. Leong P, Afrow J, Weber HP, et al. Attitudes toward patient safety standards in U.S. dental schools: a pilot study. J Dent Educ 2008;72(4):431–7.

49. Centers for Medicare & Medicaid Services. Hospital-acquired condition reduction program. Available at: https://www.cms.gov/Medicare/Medicare-Fee-for-Service-Payment/AcuteInpatientPPS/HAC-Reduction-Program.html. Accessed August 8, 2016.

50. Joint Commission. 2016 National Patient Safety Goals. Available at: https://www.jointcommission.org/standards_information/npsgs.aspx. Accessed August 8, 2016.

51. Joint Commission. Universal Protocol. Available at: https://www.jointcommission.org/standards_information/up.aspx. Accessed July 17, 2016.

52. American College of Surgeons. ACS National Surgical Quality Improvement Program. Available at: https://www.facs.org/quality-programs/acs-nsqip. Accessed August 8, 2016.

53. Fuchshuber PR, Greif W, Tidwell CR, et al. The power of the National Surgical Quality Improvement Program: achieving a zero pneumonia rate in general surgery patients. Perm J 2012;16(1):39–45.

54. Khuri SF, Henderson WG, Daley J, et al. The patient safety in surgery study: background, study design, and patient populations. J Am Coll Surg 2007;204(6):1089–102.

55. American College of Surgeons. ACS NSQIP program options. Available at: https://www.facs.org/quality-programs/acs-nsqip/program-specifics/progoptions. Accessed August 8, 2016.

56. Arce K, Moore EJ, Lohse CM, et al. The American College of Surgeons national surgical quality improvement program surgical risk calculator does not accurately predict risk of 30-day complications among patients undergoing microvascular head and neck reconstruction. J Oral Maxillofac Surg 2016;74(9):1850–8.

57. American Association of Oral and Maxillofacial Surgery. AAOMS Today, March/April 2016. Available at: http://www.aaoms.org/docs/aaoms_today/issues/2016_04.pdf. Accessed August 28, 2016.

58. Tokede O, Ramoni R, Kalenderian E. The value of checklists. J Am Dent Assoc 2014 Jul;145(7):696.

59. Walker IA, Reshamwalla S, Wilson IH. Surgical safety checklists: do they improve outcomes? Br J Anaesth 2012;109(1):47–54.

60. Joint Commission. Safe Surgery Checklist. Available at: https://www.jointcommission.org/safe_surgery_checklist/. Accessed August 8, 2016.

61. World Health Organization. WHO surgical safety checklist and implementation manual. Available at: http://www.who.int/patientsafety/safesurgery/ss_checklist/en/. Accessed August 8, 2016.

62. Haynes AB, Weiser TG, Berry WR, et al. A surgical safety checklist to reduce morbidity and mortality in a global population. N Engl J Med 2009;360:491–9.

63. de Vries EN, Hollmann MW, Smorenburg SM, et al. Development and validation of the SURgical PAtient Safety System (SURPASS) checklist. Qual Saf Health Care 2009;18:121–6.

64. de Vries EN, Prins HA, Crolla RM, et al. Effect of a comprehensive surgical safety system on patient outcomes. N Engl J Med 2010;363(20):1928–37.

65. Bock M, Fanolla A, Segur-Cabanac I, et al. A comparative effectiveness analysis of the implementation of surgical safety checklists in a tertiary care hospital. JAMA Surg 2016;151(7):639–46.

66. Christman A, Schrader S, John V, et al. Designing a safety checklist for dental implant placement: a Delphi study. J Am Dent Assoc 2014;145(2):131–40.

67. Stahel PF, Mehler PS, Clarke TJ, et al. The 5th anniversary of the "Universal Protocol": pitfalls and pearls revisited. Patient Saf Surg 2009;3(1):14.

68. Lee SL. The extended surgical time-out: does it improve quality and prevent wrong-site surgery? Perm J 2010;14(1):19–23.

69. Saufl NM. Universal protocol for preventing wrong site, wrong procedure, wrong person surgery. J Perianesth Nurs 2004;19(5):348–51.

70. Ragusa PS, Bitterman A, Auerbach B, et al. Effectiveness of surgical safety checklists in improving patient safety. Orthopedics 2016;39(2):e307–10.

71. Haugen AS, Murugesh S, Haaverstad R, et al. A survey of surgical team members' perceptions of near misses and attitudes towards time out protocols. BMC Surg 2013;13:46.

Index

Note: Page numbers of article titles are in **boldface** type.

A

Adverse drug events, in oral and maxillofacial surgery, **141–149**
  in anesthesia, 142–148
    contributing factors, 143
    improving medication safety education, 145–146
    proper management of anesthetic agents, 146–147
    proper management of emergency medication, 147–148
    reducing the incidence of, 144–145
    types of, 142–143
  definitions, 141–142
  identifying and managing, 142
  implementing a medication safety plan, 148
Adverse events, quality improvement and reporting systems for, **229–238**
Airway assessment, in preoperative planning and preparation, 134
Ambulatory oral surgery, patient safety in. See Oral and maxillofacial surgery.
Analgesia, preoperative, intraoperative, and postoperative, 136
Anesthesia, limiting medication errors and adverse drug events, **141–149**
  definitions, 141–142
  identifying and managing, 142
  implementing a medication safety plan, 148
  in oral and maxillofacial surgery, 142–148
    contributing factors, 143
    improving medication safety education, 145–146
    proper management of anesthetic agents, 146–147
    proper management of emergency medication, 147–148
    reducing the incidence of, 144–145
    types of, 142–143
  monitoring, **159–168**
    parameters and modalities of, 161–167
      circulation, 164–166
      heart rate and rhythm, 166–167
      level of consciousness, 161
      oxygenation, 161–163
      ventilation, 163–164
    pursuit of patient safety in, 160
    standards and guidelines, 160
  risks of, preoperative preparation and planning for, 137–138
  simulation training for office-based anesthesia team, **169–178**
    critical care pathways and emergency manuals, 173–174
    definition, 169–170
    emergency drills, learnings from, 171–173
    future of, 177
    impact of, 174–176
    need for office-based, 170
    roles and responsibilities, 174
    scenarios and resources for, 176–177
    as standard of care, 177
    team function, 173
    types of simulators, 170–171
Anesthetics, specific. concerns for discharge criteria, 203–204
Antibiotics, prophylactic, before surgery, 135–136
Auscultation, pretracheal, in anesthetic monitoring, 163

B

Bleeding, control of, in discharge criteria, 200–201

C

Capnography, in anesthetic monitoring, 163–164
Checklists, in quality improvement programs, 229–238
  surgical, in preventing wrong-site surgery, 155
Circulation, in anesthetic monitoring, 164–166
Colorimetric CO_2 detectors, in anesthetic monitoring, 164
Continuity of care, preoperative preparation and planning for, 138–139
Crew resource management, and patient safety, 127
Critical care pathways, in simulation training for office-based anesthesia team, 173–174

D

Diabetic patients, discharge criteria concerns after oral surgery, 204
Discharge criteria, factors impacting, after oral and maxillofacial surgery, **197–208**
  postoperative checkup, 206
  review of specific criteria, 198–203

Oral Maxillofacial Surg Clin N Am 29 (2017) 239–243
http://dx.doi.org/10.1016/S1042-3699(17)30010-9
1042-3699/17

Discharge (*continued*)
    control of bleeding, 200–201
    control of postoperative pain, 202–203
    control of vomiting/nausea, 201–202
    level of consciousness, 198–199
    postoperative instructions, 203
    stability of vital signs, 199–200
   special anesthetic concerns, 203–204
    ketamine, 204
    pharmacologic options, 204
   special patient concerns, 204–205
    diabetic patients, 204
    obstructive sleep apnea, 204–205
    pediatrics, geriatrics, and special needs
      patients, 205
   specific procedures, 205–206
   standard, 198

E

Electrical safety, and calibration of medical/surgical
   equipment, 210–212
Emergency manuals, in simulation training for office-
   based anesthesia team, 173–174
Emergency power, for patient safety, 219
Equipment safety, in oral and maxillofacial surgery,
   209–221
   back-up power and lighting, 219
   electrical safety and calibration, 210–212
   medical gases, 217–219
   radiation safety, 216–217
   sterilizer maintenance, 212–216
Errors, medical. *See* Medical errors.
Extractions. *See* Tooth extractions.

F

Fire safety, for oral and maxillofacial surgeon and
   surgical staff, **179–187**
   causes of fire, 180
   fuel sources, 180
   ignition sources, 180
   management, 184–185
   management of a fire, 182–183
   oxidizer, 180–182
   preparation, 183–184
   roles in, 183
   types of, 185–186

G

Gases, medical, safety of, 217–219
Geriatric patients, discharge criteria concerns in, 205
   preoperative preparation and planning for, 137

H

Heart rate, in anesthetic monitoring, 166–167
Heart rhythm, in anesthetic monitoring, 166–167

High-reliability organizations, 121, 127–128
   characteristics of, 128
History, medical, in preoperative planning and
   preparation, 131–132

I

Informed consent, for risk management and patient
   safety, 224–225
Intraoperative analgesia, preoperative planning
   for, 136

K

Ketamine, concerns about, in discharge criteria, 204

L

Legal issues, malpractice system and patient safety,
   223–227
   risk management impact on, 224–226
    informed consent, 224–225
    patient safety integrated into, 225–226
   torts system compared with disclosure and
    admission, 226–227
    anatomy of a malpractice claim, 226
    anatomy of disclosure and admission,
     226–227
   preventing wrong-site surgery liability claims,
    151–157
Level of consciousness, in anesthetic monitoring, 161
   in discharge criteria, 198–199
Liability. *See* Legal issues.
Lighting, back-up, for patient safety, 219

M

Malpractice system, patient safety and, **223–227**
   risk management impact on, 224–226
    informed consent, 224–225
    patient safety integrated into, 225–226
   torts system compared with disclosure and
    admission, 226–227
    anatomy of a malpractice claim, 226
    anatomy of disclosure and admission,
    226–227
Medical errors, quality improvement and reporting
   systems for, **229–238**
   root cause analysis of factors leading to, 128
Medical history, in preoperative planning and
   preparation, 131–132
Medication errors, in oral and maxillofacial surgery,
   141–149
   in anesthesia, 142–148
    contributing factors, 143
    improving medication safety education,
     145–146
    proper management of anesthetic agents,
     146–147

proper management of emergency
medication, 147–148
reducing the incidence of, 144–145
types of, 142–143
definitions, 141–142
identifying and managing, 142
implementing a medication safety plan, 148
Medication reconciliation, in preoperative planning
and preparation, 132–133
Monitoring, during anesthesia in oral and maxillofacial
surgery, **159–168**
parameters and modalities of, 161–167
circulation, 164–166
heart rate and rhythm, 166–167
level of consciousness, 161
oxygenation, 161–163
ventilation, 163–164
pursuit of patient safety in, 160
standards and guidelines, 160

N

Nausea, postoperative, in discharge criteria, 201–202
preemptive management before surgery, 134–135

O

Obstructive sleep apnea, outpatient anesthesia for
patients with, **189–196**
intraoperative management, 192
postoperative management, 192–194
criteria for discharge, 194, 204–205
medications, 193–194
rapid eye movement sleep rebound,
192–193
preoperative management, 190–192
clinical assessment, 191
overnight vs home polysomnography,
190–191
reflux and aspiration precautions, 191
STOP-BANG questionnaire for, 190
use of CPAP, 191
where to provide care, 191
Oral and maxillofacial surgery, patient safety in. See
Patient safety.
Outpatient anesthesia. See also Anesthesia.
safety in patients with obstructive sleep apnea,
189–196
Oxygenation, in anesthetic monitoring, 161–163

P

Pain control, postoperative, in discharge criteria,
202–203
preoperative, intraoperative, and postoperative,
136
Patient safety, in oral and maxillofacial surgery,
121–238

anesthesia monitoring, **159–168**
parameters and modalities of, 161–167
pursuit of patient safety in, 160
standards and guidelines, 160
discharge criteria, factors impacting, **197–208**
postoperative checkup, 206
review of specific criteria, 198–203
special anesthetic concerns, 203–204
special patient concerns, 204–205
specific procedures, 205–206
standard, 198
equipment safety, maintenance, and
inspection, **209–221**
back-up power and lighting, 219
electrical safety and calibration, 210–212
medical gases, 217–219
radiation safety, 216–217
sterilizer maintenance, 212–216
fire safety, **179–187**
causes of fire, 180
fuel sources, 180
ignition sources, 180
management, 184–185
management of a fire, 182–183
oxidizer, 180–182
preparation, 183–184
roles in, 183
types of, 185–186
general concepts, **121–129**
categories of severity of errors, 122
crew resource management, 127
high-reliability organizations, 121, 127–128
resources on, 128
root cause analysis of factors leading to
error, 128
safety culture, 127–128
simulation training, 127
systems to enhance patient safety, 126–127
types of errors in, 124
limiting medication errors and adverse drug
events, **141–149**
in anesthesia, 142–148
definitions, 141–142
identifying and managing, 142
implementing a medication safety plan, 148
malpractice system, **223–227**
risk management impact on, 224–226
torts system compared with disclosure and
admission, 226–227
obstructive sleep apnea, outpatient anesthesia
for patients with, **189–196**
intraoperative management, 192
postoperative management, 192–194
preoperative management, 190–192
preoperative preparation and planning,
131–140
airway assessment, 134

Patient (*continued*)

    continuity of care, 138–139

    in geriatric patients, 137

    medical history, 131–132

    medication reconciliation, 132–133

    pain control, 136

    in pediatric patients, 136–137

    preemptive management of nausea and vomiting, 134–135

    prophylactic antibiotics, 135–136

    risks in anesthetic management, 137–138

    tracking data, 133–134

  preventing wrong-site surgery, **151–157**

    causes of, 152–153

    preventing wrong tooth extraction, 154–157

    utility for, 153–154

  quality improvement and reporting systems, **229–238**

    assessment of safety programs, 232–234

    defining patient safety, 229–230

    external drivers of safety, 234

    future directions, 234–236

    implementing a safety program, 230–232

    promoting a safety culture, 230

  simulation training for office-based anesthesia, **169–178**

    critical care pathways and emergency manuals, 173–174

    definition, 169–170

    emergency drills, learnings from, 171–173

    future of, 177

    impact of, 174–176

    need for office-based, 170

    roles and responsibilities, 174

    scenarios and resources for, 176–177

    as standard of care, 177

    team function, 173

    types of simulators, 170–171

Pediatric patients, discharge criteria concerns in, 205

  preoperative preparation and planning for, 136–137

Planning, preoperative. *See* Preoperative preparation and planning.

Postoperative analgesia, preoperative planning for, 136

Postoperative nausea and vomiting, control of, in discharge criteria, 201–202

Power, back-up, for patient safety, 219

Preemptive management, of nausea and vomiting, 134–135

Preoperative preparation and planning, for oral and maxillofacial surgery, **131–140**

  airway assessment, 134

  continuity of care, 138–139

  in geriatric patients, 137

  medical history, 131–132

  medication reconciliation, 132–133

    pain control, 136

    in pediatric patients, 136–137

    preemptive management of nausea and vomiting, 134–135

    prophylactic antibiotics, 135–136

    risks in anesthetic management, 137–138

    tracking data, 133–134

Preparation, preoperative. *See* Preoperative preparation and planning.

Pretracheal auscultation, in anesthetic monitoring, 163

Prophylactic antibiotics, before surgery, 135–136

Pulse oximetry, in anesthetic monitoring, 161–163

Q

Quality improvement, and reporting systems in oral and maxillofacial surgery, **229–238**

  assessment of safety programs, 232–234

    benchmarking, 233–234

    self-assessment tools, 232–233

  defining patient safety, 229–230

  external drivers of safety, 234

  future directions, 234–236

  implementing a safety program, 230–232

    managing adverse events, 230–232

    minimizing risks, 230

  promoting a safety culture, 230

R

Radiation safety, of diagnostic radiation equipment, 216–217

Risk management, impact on patient safety, 224–226

  informed consent, 224–225

  patient safety integrated into, 225–226

Root cause analysis, of factors leading to errors, 128

S

Safety, patient. *See* Patient safety.

Simulation training, for office-based anesthesia team, **169–178**

  critical care pathways and emergency manuals, 173–174

  definition, 169–170

  emergency drills, learnings from, 171–173

  future of, 177

  impact of, 174–176

  need for office-based, 170

  roles and responsibilities, 174

  scenarios and resources for, 176–177

  as standard of care, 177

  team function, 173

  types of simulators, 170–171

  and patient safety, 127

Sleep apnea. *See* Obstructive sleep apnea.

Special needs patients, discharge criteria concerns in, 205
Sterilizer maintenance, for patient safety, 212–216
STOP-BANG questionnaire, preoperative, to detect obstructive sleep apnea, 190
Surgery, oral and maxillofacial, patient safety in. *See* Patient safety.
Surgical fires. *See* Fire safety.

T

Teams, simulation training for office-based anesthesia, **169–178**
    critical care pathways and emergency manuals, 173–174
    definition, 169–170
    emergency drills, learnings from, 171–173
    future of, 177
    impact of, 174–176
    need for office-based, 170
    roles and responsibilities, 174
    scenarios and resources for, 176–177
    as standard of care, 177
    team function, 173
    types of simulators, 170–171
Tooth extraction, preventing wrong-site surgery, **151–157**
    causes of, 152–153

    checklists, 155
    developing the surgical team, 154–155
    education, 154
    sign in, 155–156
    sign out, 156–157
    time out, 156
    utility for, 153–154
Torts system, compared with disclosure and admission, 226–227
    anatomy of a malpractice claim, 226
    anatomy of disclosure and admission, 226–227
Training, simulation. *See* Simulation training.

V

Ventilation, in anesthetic monitoring, 163–164
    capnography, 163–164
    direct observation, 163
    pretracheal auscultation, 163
Vital signs, stability of, in discharge criteria, 199–200
Vomiting, postoperative, in discharge criteria, 201–202
    preemptive management before surgery, 134–135

W

Wrong-site surgery. See Tooth extraction.

Moving?

Make sure your subscription moves with you!

To notify us of your new address, find your **Clinics Account Number** (located on your mailing label above your name), and contact customer service at:

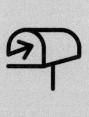

Email: journalscustomerservice-usa@elsevier.com

800-654-2452 (subscribers in the U.S. & Canada)
314-447-8871 (subscribers outside of the U.S. & Canada)

Fax number: 314-447-8029

Elsevier Health Sciences Division
Subscription Customer Service
3251 Riverport Lane
Maryland Heights, MO 63043

*To ensure uninterrupted delivery of your subscription, please notify us at least 4 weeks in advance of move.

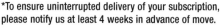

Printed and bound by CPI Group (UK) Ltd, Croydon, CR0 4YY

08/05/2025

01864699-0016